STAEHLER, ZIEGLER, VÖLTER and SCHUBERT

Color Atlas of Cytodiagnosis of the Prostate

With 117 illustrations of which
106 are in color

Color Atlas of Cytodiagnosis of the Prostate

by

W. Staehler, M. D.
Director of the Division of Urology,
University Surgical Clinic, Tübingen, Germany

H. Ziegler, M. D.
Senior Surgeon, Division of Urology,
University Surgical Clinic, Tübingen, Germany

D. Völter, M. D.
Senior Surgeon, Division of Urology,
University Surgical Clinic, Tübingen, Germany

and

G. E. Schubert, M. D.
Pathologist in Chief, Institute of Pathology,
University of Tübingen, Tübingen, Germany

Translated and Edited by

William B. Wartman, M. D.
Professor of Pathology
University of Virginia School of Medicine, Charlottesville, Va.

Distributed by

YEAR BOOK MEDICAL PUBLISHERS · INC.
35 EAST WACKER DRIVE, CHICAGO

In this book no special note has been made of drug names that are also registered trademarks. Therefore, it should not be concluded a listed drug is not patented.

All rights, especially the rights of duplication and distribution as well as of translation into foreign languages, are reserved. No part of the work may be reproduced in any form (photocopy, microfilm, or other process) without written permission of the publisher.

Original German edition Copyright© 1975 by F. K. Schattauer Verlag GmbH, Stuttgart, Germany.
Printed in Germany

Composed, printed, and bound by W. F. Mayr, Miesbach, Upper Bavaria

Library of Congress Catalog Card Number: 75–24602
ISBN 0 8151 8131 0

Preface to the English Edition

New developments in ways of looking at cells coming off the surfaces of organs – so-called exfoliative cytology – have made the diagnosis and treatment of some sorts of cancer less troublesome than before. Both carcinoma of the uterine cervix in women and carcinoma of the lung in men make this point clear. Today exfoliative cytology is generally used to make a positive diagnosis of more than one malignant neoplasm, permitting better treatment of persons in need of medical care.

In addition the use of needle aspiration biopsy has increased our ability to look into many organs that could not be biopsied before now and effectively to diagnose a possible malignant tumor. The present book gives an account, well supported by solid evidence, of the use of aspiration biopsy of the prostate using a fine needle inserted transrectally. The details of doing the biopsy and of making ready and looking at the aspirated material are given with great care and the way the cells look is made clear by a large number of color photomicrographs of the highest quality. All important diagnostic points are pictured as well as the not easily seen difficulties and possible errors that one is likely to come across. Few atlases of diagnostic cytology have as beautiful pictures as this book has and to my knowledge there are no books completely given over to the cytodiagnosis of prostatic aspiration biopsies.

It has been a pleasure to put this book into English. The only changes that have been made from the German have to do with the names of some of the drugs and therapies which have been put in harmony with American usage and current theoretical ideas. I have profited from the special knowledge of several of the persons who work in the department of pathology and I am much indebted to them for their many kindnesses. Dr. JOHN GRAYHACK, Professor of Urology, Northwestern University Medical School, has carefully gone over the clinical angles of the book and his suggestions have been of great value and are useful additions to the book.

Charlottesville, Virginia, 1976 WILLIAM B. WARTMAN, M. D.

Preface to the German Edition

Today cytodiagnosis is much used in programs for the detection of cancer. The purpose of this book is to show the practicing urologist how he can use aspiration biopsy and cytodiagnosis in his daily work, to clarify the nature of a suspicious nodule palpated in the prostate and to control the effectiveness of hormone therapy of prostatic cancer. In order to give his patients the benefit of this sort of information, it is, of course, important that the urologist be familiar with the indications for aspiration biopsy and the advantages of cytodiagnosis as well as the limitations of these practices.

It is possible to get reliable information from cytodiagnosis only when a careful technique is used for obtaining the specimen. The value of the findings is largely dependent on the experience of the operator and requires adequate time; for these reasons the procedure usually cannot be carried out in a busy general medical practice. Nevertheless, in order to provide their patients with the best possible care, it is desirable that all physicians know the advantages and limitations of the method and the meaning of the cytologic findings and be able to evaluate the report of the cytology laboratory in relation to the other clinical findings.

The goal of this book is to provide the necessary information about the technique of cytodiagnosis of aspiration biopsies of the prostate and to point out the range of its indications and the results to be expected from it.

We wish to thank Mr. K. Herzog, medical artist at the University of Tübingen, and our cytologic technologist, Miss G. Nothaft, for their help.

Our special thanks go to the publisher, F. K. Schattauer, and to Professor P. Matis for encouragement and understanding of our intentions.

It is our sincere hope that the book will make those working in cytology laboratories more interested in the special importance of cytodiagnosis for the practice of urology.

Tübingen, October 1974 *The Authors*

Table of Contents

VIII

A. Significance of Cytodiagnosis of the Prostate

Although body fluids have been examined occasionally by cytologic methods since the middle of the last century, it is only since the basic investigations of Papanicolaou that regular cytodiagnosis has become a reality. To be sure, his first contribution in 1928 on the detection of suspected carcinoma cells in vaginal smears found no general acceptance. However, his monograph published with Traut in 1943 rapidly brought about acceptance of cytodiagnosis as a useful clinical tool.[17] The success of exfoliative cytology in the diagnosis of carcinoma of the female genitalia raised the hope that the method might also be useful in the early discovery of carcinoma of the prostate. However, the first enthusiasm of most investigators soon diminished in view of the fact that only about 40% of patients with early cancer of the prostate could be discovered by examining smears of prostatic fluid.[14] The good results obtained with exfoliative cytology in carcinoma of the uterine cervix were not obtained in carcinoma of the prostate. This is understandable because in cervical carcinoma a smear of a suspicious lesion can be taken under direct vision, but in the case of the prostate only nonspecific secretion can be collected for cytologic examination. As a consequence of this nonspecificity of the sample, it is impossible to obtain the desired accuracy of diagnosis in early prostatic carcinoma by this method.

Aspiration biopsy gives us another way of getting material for diagnosis. As opposed to exfoliative cytology in which cells for examination are obtained either from the surface or from cells spontaneously shed in body fluids or washed from the body by irrigation, cells are aspirated by a very thin needle used to puncture a specific area. This method, first described in 1930 by Ferguson for the diagnosis of tumors of the prostate, has made possible cytologic investigation of organs that do not naturally shed their cells. Use of the fine-needle technique also eliminates the occurrence of the complications that may occur with a punch biopsy (Tru-Cut or Vim-Silverman needle), which is needed for a histologic sample. Ferguson's technique for aspiration biopsy using a fine needle inserted through the perineum and cytologic examination of the aspirate was improved in 1960 by Franzén and his colleagues, who developed transrectal aspiration biopsy of the prostate.[4,6] By means of such a direct approach to the prostate the accuracy of the cytologic method was greatly increased. Thus we now have a reliable, simple, low-risk and practical method of getting material for cytologic examina-

1

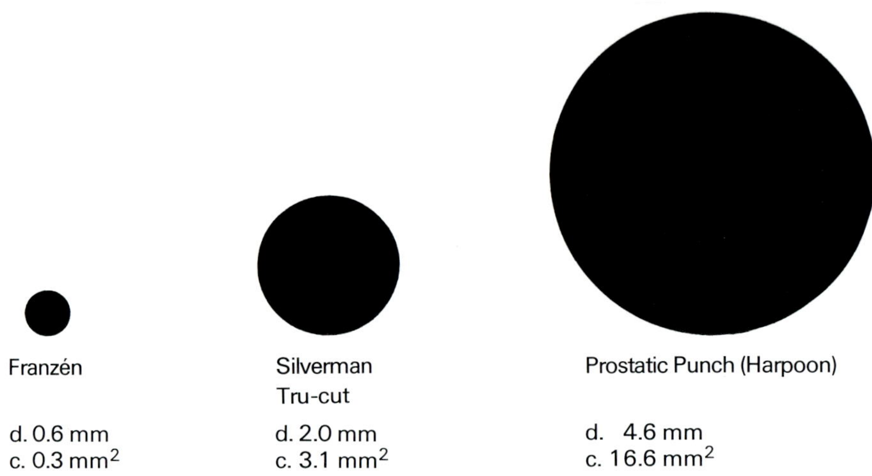

Fig.A.1. – Commonly used biopsy needles seen in cross section (*d*, diameter, *c*, cross-sectional surface).

tion which can be used on ambulatory patients who need not have much preoperative preparation.[1] Figure A.1 shows the comparative diameters of the Franzén needle, the Tru-Cut or Vim-Silverman needle, and the prostatic punch, which are respectively 0.6 mm, 2 mm, and 4.6 mm and have cross-sectional surfaces that are of the ratio 1:11:50.[25] It is quite clear that complications may be expected chiefly when a large needle is used.

Franzén's method aims at getting the same results for suspected prostatic tumors as have been obtained by using exfoliative cytology for suspected carcinoma of the uterine cervix in women. In addition, aspiration biopsy instead of the examination of individual exfoliated dead cells yields groups of living cells, which are easier to evaluate. This technique now makes it possible to diagnose carcinoma of the prostate with the same degree of accuracy as for cervical carcinoma. Experience has shown that in the case of carcinoma of the uterine cervix, the diagnostic accuracy in the hands of competent observers is between 90 and 95%.

According to Faul, Klosterhalfen, and Schmiedt,[7] the accuracy of diagnosing prostatic carcinoma with fine-needle aspiration biopsy is 92%. In order to double check this claim we have investigated 190 patients with prostatic carcinoma by means of simultaneously performed cytodiagnosis and histologic biopsy.[19] We found that the two methods agreed in 97% of the cases. In only one patient (0.2%) was an existing carcinoma undiscovered by cytologic examination and in only five patients (2.6%) was a carcinoma that had been diagnosed by cytology unconfirmed by histology. However, this number of false diagnoses by cytology may be misleading since histologic diagnosis by harpoon biopsy does not always detect a small carcinoma.[18]

Because a very good sample may be obtained by Franzén's technique of transrectal aspiration biopsy using a fine needle, prostatic cytodiagnosis has come to have the same degree of accuracy as the ordinary histologic biopsy for the diagnosis of prostatic carcinoma.[7] Therefore, we use a punch biopsy for histologic study only in cases of cytologic problems or before radical prostatectomy. Not only is aspiration biopsy better than a perineal punch for obtaining a satisfactory biopsy sample, but it is also better for the patient. The advantages of the aspiration biopsy come from the use of a very fine needle that is thinner than a No. 14 hypodermic needle. It makes possible direct transrectal puncture of the prostate in patients without previous preparation and allows a biopsy to be taken directly from a suspicious area. By puncturing the prostate in a wide fan-shaped area, the chances of hitting the lesion can be much increased. There is almost no attendant pain, and because of the very slight trauma, complications such as late bleeding or attacks of fever seldom occur.[15] In 1,020 patients from whom we took prostatic aspiration biopsies with the Franzén needle, we encountered fever as high as 39°C for 1–2 days in nine patients (0.9%). Fifteen patients (1.5%) stated that they had slightly bloody urine on the first micturition after the aspiration biopsy. We have not observed any other complications.[22]

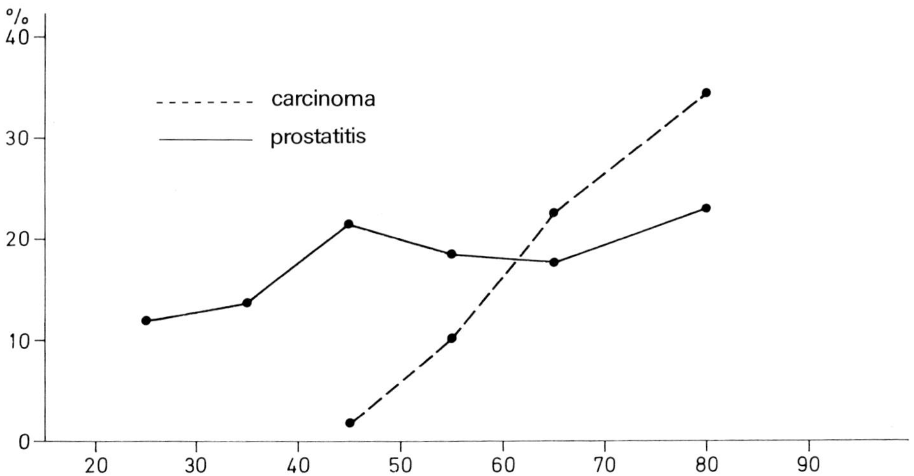

Fig. A.2. — Percentage age frequency of prostatitis and prostatic carcinoma in aspiration biopsies of 1,187 patients grouped in ten-year intervals.

In contrast to gynecologic cytodiagnosis, which is based on examination of exfoliated cells and where routine examination is practical in all cancer detection examinations, we use fine-needle aspiration biopsy of the prostate only when the suspicion of tumor is well founded, usually after digital rectal examination. Therefore, it is essential to do a rectal examination routinely in every cancer detection examination in men over 45 years of age.[1,21] All nodules or areas of abnormal consistency should be suspected of being either a carcinoma, a specific or nonspecific inflammation, or a stone. In order to exclude carcinoma, an aspiration biopsy is performed on every palpable prostatic nodule. Since not every palpable prostatic nodule is necessarily a carcinoma, it is essential to examine every nodule by either histologic or cytologic biopsy before treatment is started.[20]

Figure A.2 compares the percentage frequency of prostatitis and prostatic carcinoma in various age groups as diagnosed by cytologic methods.[23] The curves are based on 1,187 patients in whom an aspiration biopsy was carried out because of suspicious findings on rectal palpation of the prostate. From the fourth to the fifth decade the curve shows an almost linear frequency of prostatic carcinoma as a cause of suspicious rectal findings. By the sixtieth year the chances are about equal of a suspicious rectal lesion being due to either carcinoma or prostatitis, whereas in older age groups carcinoma is the chief cause of a palpable nodule. Because it is not possible to diagnose the nature of a nodule by rectal palpation alone, any induration of the prostate is an absolute indication for an aspiration biopsy.

The technique of transrectal aspiration biopsy developed by Franzén is not only of value for the cytodiagnosis of the presence or absence of a prostate carcinoma. It is also used for the cytodiagnosis of the grade of malignancy and for assessing the adequacy of hormone therapy of a carcinoma.[10] On the basis of the cytologic picture, it is possible to decide the grade of malignancy of a prostatic carcinoma, which has great prognostic value when considered with the clinical findings.[5]

Fifteen to 20% of patients with prostatic carcinoma do not respond to estrogen therapy. The typical degenerative changes that occur in carcinoma cells during treatment with estrogens are easily detected by cytologic studies,[19] and if these changes fail to develop it can be assumed that the cancer is hormone resistant. The treatment can then be changed without great loss of time.

The difficulties that surround the diagnosis of prostatitis are well known. Often the diagnosis can neither be established nor excluded on clinical grounds. In such patients an aspiration biopsy makes possible an accurate differential diagnosis and a proper plan of treatment.[24]

4

Transrectal aspiration biopsy of the prostate by Franzén's method has by now been established as a simple and reliable technique. It is a routine mode of action—like cytologic investigation of vaginal and cervical smears in gynecology—and has a definite place in any program of cancer detection in men.

Because of the improvement in technique, prostatic cytology is no longer inferior in accuracy to histologic methods. On account of the slight trauma incurred in obtaining an aspiration biopsy, cytologic study of the prostate in our opinion is the method of choice for cancer detection.

B. Technique

1. Sampling

a) Prostatic Secretion

Controversy still exists over the value of examining prostatic secretion for the diagnosis of carcinoma of the prostate. Secretion obtained by rectal prostatic massage cannot be identified with certainty as coming from the urethra, seminal vesicles, or prostate, and occasionally no fluid at all can be obtained because of decreased glandular function or obstruction of the excretory ducts. Therefore, exfoliative cytology of the prostate does not have the diagnostic reliability that it does, for example, in the diagnosis of cervical carcinoma in women in whom a suspicious lesion can be sampled under direct vision.[11, 12]

Cytologic examination of prostatic secretion in suspected prostatic carcinoma is thus unreliable for making a definitive diagnosis. On the whole, cytologic examination of prostatic secretion is meaningful only in cases where a nodule cannot be palpated and there is thus no indication for an aspiration biopsy. In these circumstances there are very few cases in which it is possible to make an early diagnosis of prostatic carcinoma.

b) Aspiration Biopsy

Aspiration biopsy provides a sample of living cells from a suspicious lesion. It is not, however, useful in a screening program for cancer detection. It is rightly used where a suspicion of cancer is well founded, as for example by the discovery on rectal examination of a palpable nodule or a prostate of unusual consistency. In such cases, use of the fine-needle technique allows direct sampling of the suspicious area through the rectum in ambulatory patients and without preoperative preparation. Such targeted sampling is not possible by sharp perineal biopsy.

The current technique of transrectal aspiration biopsy of the prostate using a fine needle was described by Franzén in 1960. Without previous preparation of the patient, a very fine needle is inserted into the prostate and cellular material is sucked into a syringe screwed to the needle. The punctate is then smeared on a microscopic slide and

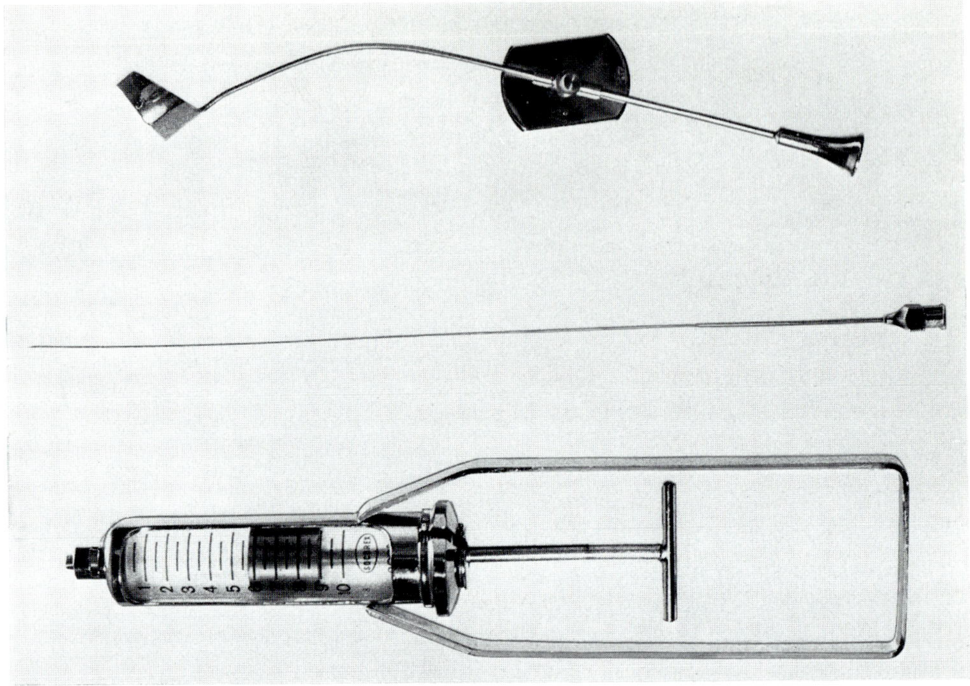

Fig. B.1. – Franzén equipment for aspiration biopsy, consisting of syringe, needle, and needle guide.

examined cytologically. Only a needle, a needle guide, and a syringe are needed (Fig. B.1).

A special grip on the instrument makes it possible to hold the aspiration syringe in one hand while the other hand holds the needle guide and with the index finger guides the needle to the place in the prostate from which the sample will be taken. Before the puncture is made, the syringe should be tested for tightness and the needle then screwed on the syringe. To obtain a good specimen the syringe must be quickly withdrawn and quickly released to the starting position again. If this is not done the specimen may become coated with silicon. The aspiration needle is 20 cm long and has a thick end piece and a very thin shaft. The needle must be washed with water immediately after use in order to keep the lumen open. Because the thin shaft of the needle is exactly the same length as the needle guide, the transition from the thick end piece to the thin portion can be used as a marker. When the thick part of the needle enters the funnel of the needle guide, the point of the needle will have entered the tissue.

8

The curved needle guide adjusts easily to the palpating finger. The proximal end is funnel shaped so that the puncture needle can be introduced without trouble. The distal end of the needle guide forms a ring through which the point of the needle protrudes. This ring is split on the dorsal side so that the index finger can be readily inserted. Near the middle of the needle guide is a movable metal plate that fits well in the palm of the hand, and a screw allows it to be fixed in the best position.

Before each use the whole apparatus is cleaned and sterilized. Sterile precautions are necessary to avoid possible introduction of pathogenic organisms against which the patient may have no resistance. The patient is now put in the lithotomy position—as if for cytoscopy. After putting on a glove, the left index finger—on a right-handed person—is inserted into the metal ring of the needle guide and a rubber finger cot is pulled over the metal ring and the index finger. The metal plate of the needle guide is now pressed against the palm of the hand with the third and fourth fingers, while the thumb and the index finger are extended (Fig. B.2). To avoid aspiration of lubricant into the needle, which lies on the ventral side, only the dorsal side of the finger is lubricated. Thus prepared, the needle guide, which lies on the lubricated left index finger, can be inserted into the rectum and the suspicious area palpated once again. Now the aspira-

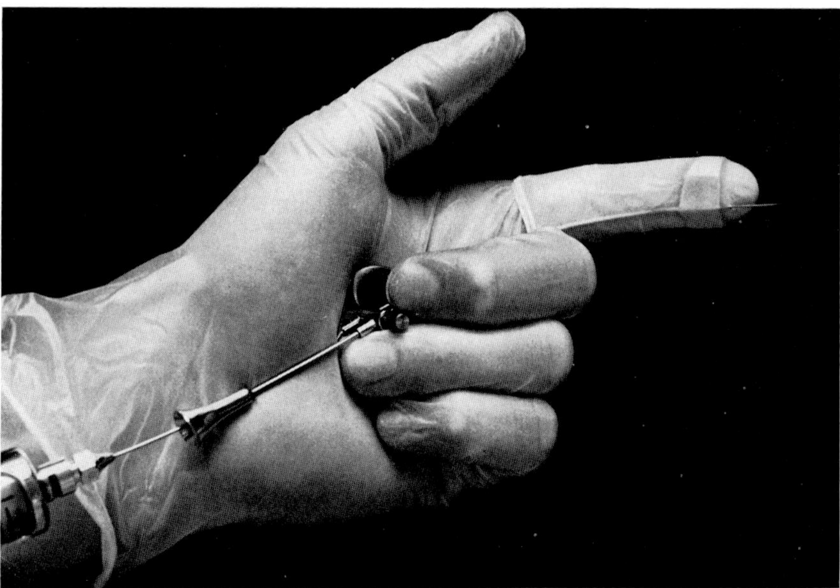

Fig. B.2. – The aspiration needle assembly of Franzén held in the left hand. The thick end of the aspiration needle is in place in the funnel of the needle guide. The point of the needle has left the ring of the needle guide and perforated the rubber finger on the end of the index finger.

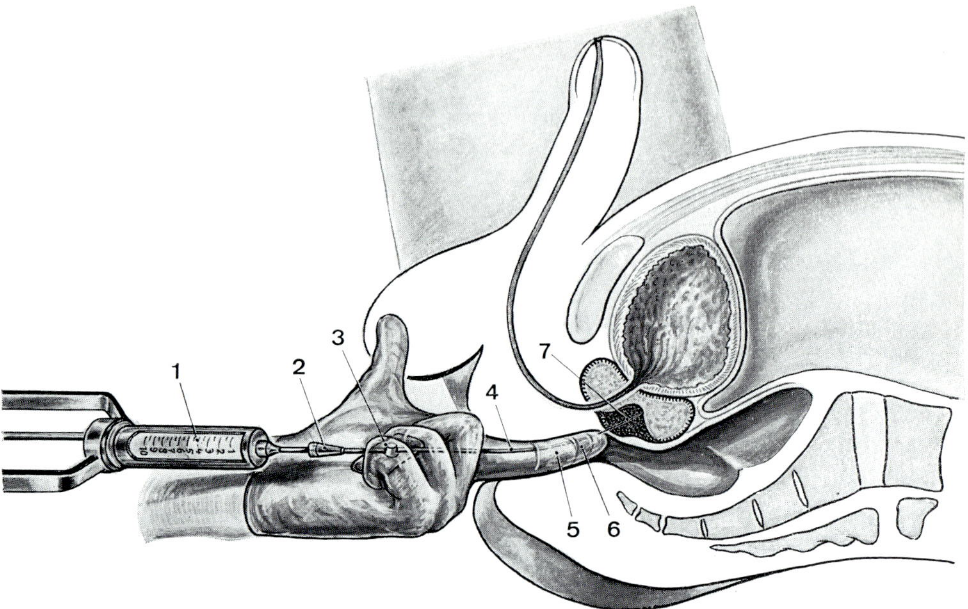

Fig. B.3. — Schematic drawing of the anatomic relations during transrectal aspiration with a fine needle according to Franzén. *1,* aspiration syringe, *2,* funnel-shaped end of the needle guide, *3,* fixation plate of the needle guide, *4,* needle guide, *5,* rubber finger over the needle guide, *6,* end ring of the needle guide, *7,* puncture needle.

tion syringe with the previously attached needle is taken in the right hand and inserted into the funnel-shaped end of the needle guide and pushed forward until the point lies even with the part of the needle guide that is in the rectum (Fig. B.3). The barely protruding point of the needle is guided by the palpating left index finger and placed over the suspicious area of the prostate. The right hand then advances the needle exactly 5 to 10 mm. All is now ready to aspirate and the plunger of the syringe may be pulled back. Under the vacuum created, the right hand slides the aspiration needle back and forth six or seven times for a distance of 5 to 10 mm. In this way cellular material is aspirated. At the conclusion of the puncture, the plunger is released in order to break the vacuum, and only now should the needle be withdrawn from the prostate. The left index finger with the needle guide remains in the rectum. In taking the needle out of the prostate, care must be taken to free the plunger of the syringe, as the loss of pressure will draw the sample from the needle into the cylinder of the syringe, thus losing much of the sample. Moreover, rectal contents will be drawn into the needle and the remaining aspirate is usually unusable. Therefore, it is very important to release the plunger of the

10

syringe while removing the needle from the prostate. Usually the aspirated sample is then in the needle and not in the syringe.

The syringe with the needle unscrewed is then handed to an assistant who removes the needle from the syringe and draws back the plunger to fill the syringe with air. The air-filled syringe is reattached to the needle that still contains the biopsy specimen. By pressing on the plunger of the syringe, the biopsy specimen is squirted from the needle onto one end of a labeled microscopic slide. Using a second slide, the aspirated material is smeared just like a blood smear, air dried (Fig. B. 4), and later stained with May-Grünwald-Giemsa. The assistant now returns the syringe with the needle attached to the surgeon, who does a second and third puncture. During the course of these procedures, the left index finger of the surgeon with the needle guide is kept in the rectum. At the end of the procedure, first the biopsy needle and then the needle guide are withdrawn from the rectum. In carcinoma the cells in the aspirated biopsy because of their decreased adhesiveness are usually more abundant than are the cells in a case of nodular hyperplasia.[2, 5] If the puncture has gone too deep, urine will be aspirated and this is useless for cytologic examination. When this happens the urine is expressed from the needle and the suspicious area is punctured again.

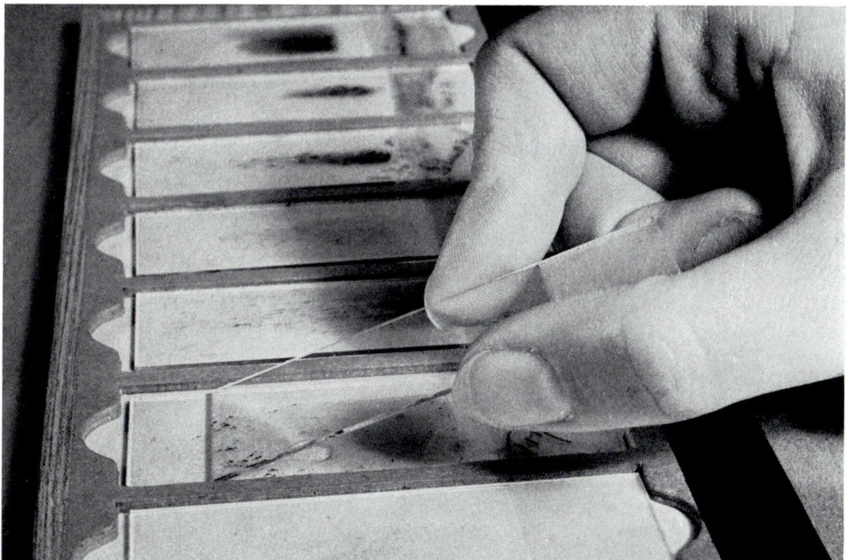

Fig. B.4. — Smearing the aspirated cellular material with the aid of a second microscopic slide. The ground glass end of the slide is labeled with a pencil, and the prepared slides are placed in a slide case and sent to the cytology laboratory.

c) Fixation and Shipment of Biopsy Smears

We regularly use air-dried, unfixed material stained with May-Grünwald-Giemsa for prostatic cytology. The smeared microscopic slide without any further fixing is sent to the cytology laboratory. A lapse of two to four days between taking the aspiration biopsy and staining the slide is of no consequence. Only when there is a delay of more than four days should a fixative be used. For this purpose a ready-made spray fixative (e. g., Pro-Fix) is useful. Because the smear must be fixed while it is still moist, the slide is sprayed with the fixative immediately after smearing the aspirated material. If inadvertently the smear is partly dried by the air, the ease of interpretation is considerably reduced.

The moist smear is fixed by spraying it three or four times from a distance of about 20 cm. The smear is then dried in the air for about 10 minutes, after which it may be shipped without further handling. Before staining, the fixed preparation must be immersed in either distilled water or 50% alcohol to moisten the fixative. With Papanicolaou's stain it is essential to fix the smear first.

The labeled microscopic slides (best done with pencil on the ground glass end) are sent to the cytology laboratory in a suitable container along with instructions and the patient's pertinent data, including the findings on rectal examination, the clinical diagnosis, and any contemplated hormone treatment.

2. Staining Methods[15]

Unstained aspirated cells, like exfoliated cells, are almost invisible in the light microscope. Various staining methods are therefore used to make the cells visible and to detect variation in intensity of staining in different parts of the smear. The optimal method of staining a smear is a personal matter. Each stain produces an acceptable cellular picture and the choice is dependent on the experience and preference of the observer.

We prefer May-Grünwald-Giemsa stain because it can be used on unfixed, air-dried preparations. The staining process takes a relatively short time and the stain gives a very good picture of the distribution of the nuclear chromatin. In addition, in unfixed, air-dried smears there is little distortion of cells and nuclei due to shrinkage.

Because critical examination of the cell nucleus is essential in prostatic cytology, the ratio of nucleus to cytoplasm is less important, and cytoplasmic changes are of scant value, this method of staining is completely satisfactory. Characteristic nuclear changes in prostatic carcinoma cells, such as the frequent, large, prominent nucleoli, are clearly seen. However, certain other stains, such as hematoxylin-eosin and Papanicolaou, may be useful for investigating special questions. We use these stains only to supplement the May-Grünwald-Giemsa stain.

The chief differences between the May-Grünwald-Giemsa stain and the Papanicolaou stains are the cytoplasmic monochromasia and the clear differentiation of cells in the former. In unfixed, air-dried smears stained with May-Grünwald-Giemsa, the cells essentially retain their natural size.

Hematoxylin-eosin (HE) stain is used mostly for histologic sections and by pathologist-cytologists, since it displays well both the nucleus and the cytoplasm and the pathologist is familiar with this stain. Contrasted with May-Grünwald-Giemsa, there arc only slight differences. Thus, with HE the internal structure of the nucleus is slightly paler and the cell borders are more clearly seen (Fig. B.5).

Below are given the different steps in the various staining methods as we use them for prostatic cytology.

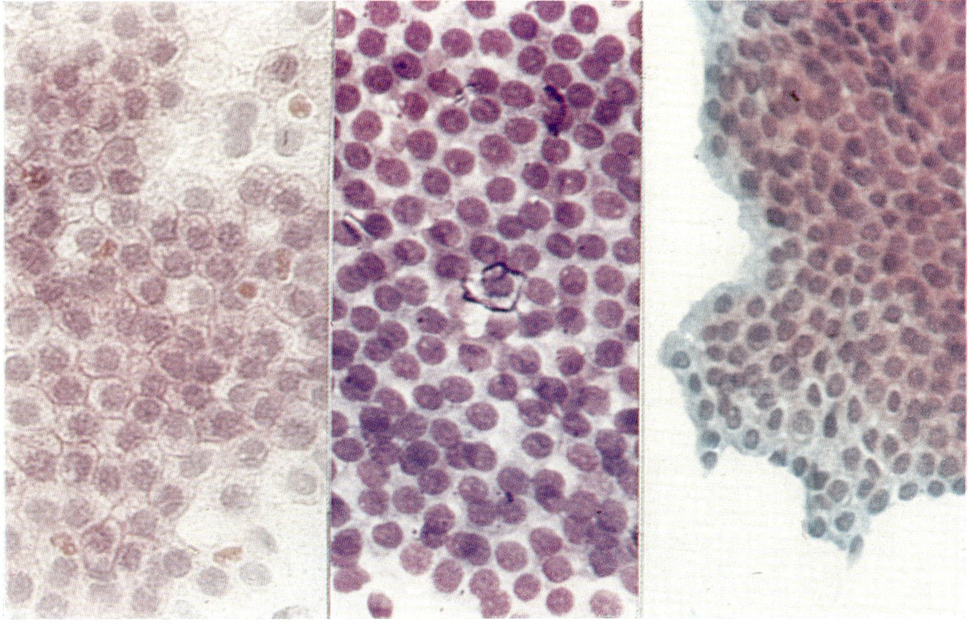

Fig. B.5. — Comparison of different stains of the same aspirate from a case of nodular hyperplasia (adenoma) of the prostate. *Left,* Hematoxylin-eosin; *middle,* May-Grünwald-Giemsa; *right,* Papanicolaou (each 250×).

May-Grünwald-Giemsa Stain

Unfixed, air-dried smears

    1. May-Grünwald solution, modified
       (Eosin-methylene blue solution, Merck 1424) . . . . 4–5 minutes
    2. Distilled water . . . . 4–5 minutes
    3. Giemsa solution (1 ml Giemsa in 10 ml tap water)
       (azur-eosin-methylene blue solution, Merck 9204) . . . . 18–20 minutes
    4. Rinse in distilled water
    5. Air dry
    6. Xylol
    7. Cover with Permount or the like

HE Stain (Hematoxylin-Eosin)

Air-dried, unfixed smears

    1. Fix in 96% alcohol . . . . 15 minutes to maximum of 48 hours
    2. Mayers hematoxylin . . . . 12 minutes
    3. Rinse in running water . . . . 10 minutes
    4. 1% eosin solution . . . . 2–3 minutes
    5. Distilled water . . . . about 10 times
    6. 70% alcohol . . . . about 10 times
    7. 96% alcohol . . . . 5 minutes
    8. Absolute alcohol . . . . 5 minutes
    9. Xylol . . . . 5 minutes to maximum of 1 hour
   10. Cover with Permount

If the smears have been fixed with spray fixative, wash it off with distilled water or
50% alcohol and start with step 2.

Papanicolaou Stain

For moist smears fixed with spray fixative. After washing with distilled water or
50% alcohol:

    1. Harris hematoxylin . . . . 6 minutes
    2. Distilled water
    3. 0.25% HCl-alcohol . . . . 6 times
    4. Running water . . . . 6 minutes
    5. Distilled water
    6. 50% alcohol

7. 70% alcohol
8. 80% alcohol
9. 95% alcohol
10. Orange G 6 (Merck 6887) .... 1.5 minutes
11. 95% alcohol
12. 95% alcohol
13. EA 50 (Merck 9272) .... 1.5 minutes
14. 95% alcohol
15. 95% alcohol
16. 95% alcohol
17. Absolute alcohol
18. Absolute alcohol
19. Xylol
20. Cover with Permount or the like

3. Microscopy

A full account of the microscope and its various attachments is outside the scope of this book and only some practical hints are given for using the microscope in prostatic cytodiagnosis.

a) Light Microscopy

For routine diagnostic work with transmitted light, a microscope with built-in illumination is most useful, especially if the work is prolonged. A dual viewing microscope with a built-in pointer through which two observers can look at the same time eases the task of teaching students and is an aid in discussing specific observations.

Objectives. — The objectives are mounted in a revolving head situated in the lower end of the microscope tube. Planar objectives are especially helpful in cytologic work because the entire field is sharp all the way out to the edge. Apochromates with optimal correction give the best color rendition of the preparation and are preferred by most cytologists. The objectives most used are those with magnifications of 2.5, 6.3, 10, 16, 25, 40, and 100. We regularly use a 10× scouting lens for the first look at the slide and then 25× and 40× objectives for detailed examination. The manufacturer gives the most important properties of the lens on each objective. For example, Plan 40/0.65;

160/0.17 means that this objective produces a plane field of vision and a magnification of 40. The number 0.65 indicates the numerical aperture, which measures the quantity of light rays that pass through the angle of the aperture. The resolving power of the objective is determined by this aperture. For optimal results the total magnification should be 500–1,000 times the aperture so that the objective will completely resolve the individual elements of the picture for the eye. This total magnification is calculated by multiplying the magnification of the objective by that of the ocular. For example, it is not appropriate to use an ocular of more than 16× with a 40× objective having an aperture of 0.65 (40×16 = 640×0.65 = 650), since with this ocular only a small part of the image formed by the objective can be observed. Objectives of higher resolution have an aperture over 1.0, and in order to utilize their full potential resolution oil immersion must be used. Oil immersion lenses with 100× magnification, for example, require an aperture between 1.00 and 1.4 and the introduction of a fluid optically similar to glass between the surface of the microscopic slide and the front lens of the objective. This procedure eliminates the bending of the light beam by the layer of air lying between the slide and the lens of the objective, and thus it considerably improves the performance of the microscope. Purified, thick cedar oil (n_D=1.515) is usually used.

The number 160 given on the objective in the above example is the length of the tube of the microscope (only of importance when interchanging individual parts of different microscopes); 0.17 is the ideal thickness of the slide in millimeters, which must be more exactly met the greater the magnification of the objective.

Condenser. — In order to take maximal advantage of the aperture of a high-power objective, a condenser is placed beneath the objective in the path of the light beam. In principle the structure of this condenser is the reverse of that of the objective so that entering parallel light rays are spread out in a wide cone and illuminate as much as possible of the specimen under examination. The aperture number of the condenser may also be indicated on it. For most work an aperture of 0.9 is enough. For accurate reproduction of color it is best to use an achromatic-aplanar condenser with an aperture of 1.3–1.14, which ideally should be immersed in oil between the upper surface of the condenser and the undersurface of the microscopic slide.

Ocular. — Oculars are designated as simple orthoscopic oculars or compensating plano-oculars. The former are unsuitable for achromatic objectives. We prefer a combination of compensating plano-oculars with planochromatic objectives since they correct simultaneously for flatness and color. Customarily, 8, 10, and 12.5×, wide-angle oculars are used to facilitate rapid survey of a slide.

Filters. – For routine examination of prostatic cytology with artificial light, we use a pale blue filter which gives a color image similar to daylight. A green filter is used when it is desired to emphasize cell margins (see Fig. D.5).

Mechanical Stage. – A mechanical stage makes possible systematic examination of the entire smear, and a Vernier scale along one side of it allows the position of any spot in the slide to be noted and relocated.

Köhler's Method of Illumination with Transmitted Light

The slide is placed on the stage of the microscope with the smear or cover glass side up. The light is adjusted to an agreeable degree of intensity either by regulating the light-dimmer switch or by using a filter. The binoculars are adjusted until there is a single field of vision. The eye distance is read on the round scale between the oculars and the same number is set on the ocular socket, thereby correcting for distances between the two eyes of different persons.

Using a medium power lens (10× or 16× objective), focus the smear sharply.

Open widely the light diaphragm in the base of the microscopy and partly close the condenser diaphragm.

Slowly rack down the condenser from its highest possible position until the margins of the light condenser are sharp and appear as a small circle of bright light.

Center this bright circular image of the light diaphragm by turning the centering screws in the condenser holder.

Now open the light diaphragm until it exactly overlaps the field of vision. If the visual field is now not evenly illuminated, it will be necessary to adjust the light bulb in its socket.

Close the aperture diaphragm in the condenser until maximum contrast is obtained in the field of vision (about 1/5–1/3 closed).

This sort of careful preparation of the microscope is necessary in order to get the best possible microscopic images.

b) Phase Contrast Microscopy

When observed with transmitted light, unstained cells absorb little light and give an image that is scarcely recognizable and poor in contrast. It is for this reason that we customarily stain the cells with various dyes. However, with the use of phase contrast microscopy unstained, viable cells can be easily studied.

The principle of the method rests upon the following phenomenon: very little or no light is absorbed in its passage through fresh, unstained cells; that is, its amplitude is not diminished, but the light is slightly delayed in passing through the various cell structures and so there is a slight dislocation of its phase. This delayed arrival of single rays on the other side of the objective, the "phase difference",cannot be recognized by the eye. However, by placing an interference in the path of the light ray the phase difference can be changed to an amplitude difference, therefore to a light-dark difference that the eye can recognize. In a phase contrast adaptor, such a change is made in the condenser and objective. Images of great contrast are produced so that it is possible to distinguish clearly the cellular detail in living cells and to differentiate between normal cells and tumor cells.

The phase contrast microscope has long been used in cytologic research, but in most laboratories at the present time it is little used for routine cytodiagnosis. However, in the future this may become a useful rapid method of prostatic cytodiagnosis.

c) Fluorescence Microscopy

In fluorescence microscopy, fixed material is labeled with certain yellow or red dyes that fluoresce when examined in short-wave, ultraviolet light. This property of certain substances, the so-called fluorochromes, depends upon their ability to give up a portion of their energy supply as light of long wave length when irradiated with ultraviolet light. The fluorochrome most used in cytology is acridine orange. In the usual fluorescence equipment, a high-pressure mercury vapor lamp produces the energizing light. An energy filter is put in the light path in front of the objective that permits the short-wave portion to pass through but interrupts unwanted long-wave green and orange components. A blocking filter between objective and eye absorbs the short-wave rays and allows only those waves to pass that are produced in the specimen by the fluorescent light. This filter must be carefully placed in order to prevent retinal injury by the intense ultraviolet light.

Normal prostatic cells do not fluoresce, but by coating them with fluorochrome they can be visualized in the fluorescent microscope as fluorescing bright objects (see Figs. D.19, D.75). Groups of cells are very easily found this way. The stain is used particularly for displaying the green fluorescence of DNA and the red of RNA in ultraviolet light. However, the method is not as good for demonstrating cytologic details of individual cells as is examination of stained cells by transmitted light. For this reason, fluorescence microscopy is not yet an accepted procedure for routine cytodiagnosis.

18

Nevertheless, since fluorochrome can be used to label antibodies in immunohistology, it may well be possible in the future to undertake immunological studies that may open a whole new field of investigation.

d) Electron microscopy

Use of sedimentation and filtration techniques now makes it possible to concentrate the cells obtained from an aspiration biopsy sufficiently to embed them for electron microscopy. In addition, the scanning electron microscope permits three-dimensional images of smeared cells and opens up new possibilities for fundamental research. For the present, however, relatively few laboratories are equipped to use these methods.

C. General Cytology

1. Structure of the Normal Cell

Epithelial cells of the prostate glands have round, relatively small nuclei which lie typically in the middle of the cells. In dried smears, the nucleoplasm has a loose appearance and frequently there are small nucleoli which may be numerous. Mitoses are rare. For the most part, the cytoplasm is finely granular. Vacuoles are seen in both the cytoplasm and the nucleus and are caused largely either by the air drying or by osmotic cytolysis resulting from simultaneously aspirated urine.

In adults there are no striking variations in the nuclear-cytoplasmic relation, but in children there may be great variation. In prostatic cytology, we are interested not only in evaluating individual cells but also in noting the adhesion of the sheets of prostatic cells that are always present in normal smear preparations. These sheets, which are made up of a monolayer of epithelial cells derived from the cells lining the glandular lumens, are detached from the basement membrane in more or less large sheets by the suction of the aspiration. Such "wallpaper shreds" have characteristic forms and may consist of a dozen or even a thousand adherent cells. The cells in these sheets show a striking uniformity, especially of the nuclei, and frequently a normal prostatic smear can be recognized with the low-power lens (100×).

Only rarely are cells or nuclei found that have become separated from the sheet, and such cells should always be examined most carefully to determine if they have come from the cell sheet or are cells aspirated incidentally from neighboring organs or, most importantly, show features of malignancy. Such detached cells have a "decoy" function and when they are seen, every slide must be carefully examined for possible malignancy. At times homogeneous granules are seen irregularly but diffusely superimposed on the sheets of cells and in the background of the smear. The origin and composition of these granules are still unknown.

Cytologic smears of young persons can be difficult to diagnose because of their great nuclear polymorphism and the dissociation of cells from the sheets even though there are no other evidences of malignancy. Knowledge of the age of the patient is important therefore, and may help to avoid making a grossly false report.

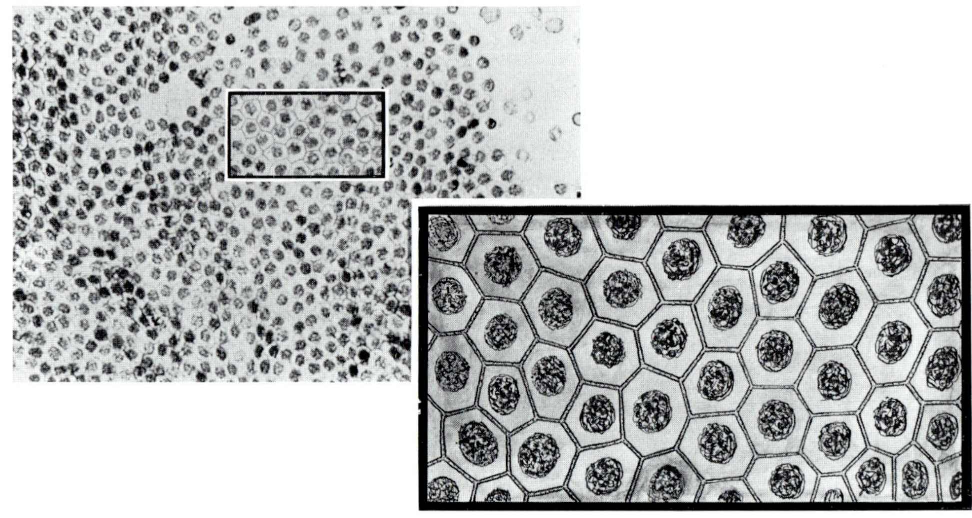

Fig. C.1. — Schematic representation of a sheet of normal prostatic cells with regular cells, having round, centrally placed, loose appearing nuclei and honeycomb arrangement of cell borders.

In nodular hyperplasia (adenoma) of elderly patients, the cytologic smear shows an orderly, regular sheet pattern and the most uniform cellular picture of any age group. Most of the cell borders are polygonal and six sided (Fig. C.1).

2. Inflammation

Cytologically, prostatitis may show all the signs of inflammation without there being concomitant clinical evidence.

Acute prostatitis, which can result in an abscess in severe cases, cytologically shows neutrophilic granulocytes almost exclusively. Prostatic cells become detached, lose their sheet arrangement, and are infiltrated and surrounded by leukocytes with segmented nuclei. This inflammatory exudate lessens the transparency of the preparation.

Frequently, however, there is an acute episode of chronic recurrent inflammation in which all kinds of granulocytes and lymphocytes are seen, depending on the severity, as well as histiocytes, monocytes, and plasma cells. Usually it is possible to distinguish between subacute and chronic prostatitis or an acute exacerbation of the latter. In prostatitis, the prostatic cells mainly show degenerative nuclear changes, such as swel-

22

ling, polychromasia, netlike clumping of chromatin, vacuole formation, pyknosis, and condensation of the nucleolus, and the condition may be very difficult to distinguish from malignancy.

In such cases it may be best to make a provisional diagnosis and to treat the patient with antibiotics for 6–8 weeks and then take a second biopsy. In most cases, the degenerative changes caused by the inflammation will have disappeared and it will be easier to evaluate the biopsy and to exclude or confirm the diagnosis of carcinoma.

Granulomatous prostatitis is an infrequently encountered form of specific prostatic inflammation. Besides histiocytes, there are multinucleated giant cells, great numbers of plasma cells, and scattered eosinophilic granulocytes. The granuloma formation produces hard, palpable nodules mimicking cancer and can be diagnosed certainly only by biopsy. However, because a carcinoma can arise in granulomatous prostatitis, another biopsy should be taken after a three-month interval.

Tuberculous prostatitis cytologically shows expanding necrosis.

3. Carcinoma

All the general cytologic features of malignancy are used to diagnose carcinoma of the prostate: loss of uniform cell pattern together with polymorphism that exceeds normal limits of both cells and nuclei. Hyperchromatism is discovered only occasionally and for the most part in pyknotic, bizarre nuclei.

Frequently the nucleoli are increased in size and number and may account for one-seventh to one-third of the nuclear mass. The discovery of such nucleoli is pathognomonic of carcinoma. Shifting of the nuclear-cytoplasmic ratio in favor of the nucleus is seen chiefly in poorly differentiated carcinomas, whereas undifferentiated carcinomas show mostly pathologic nuclei. Changes in the cell pattern of the aggregates are decisive in making a diagnosis of malignancy. Usually a greater number of cells are aspirated from carcinomatous than from normal tissue, a fact explained by the decreased adhesiveness of tumor cells.[3, 16] Usually tumor smears are also free of blood whereas erythrocytes are frequently found in smears of normal cells. With a good smear technique, the large amount of material makes it possible to evaluate the cells, the degree of aggregation as shown by the formation of adherent sheets, the effects of squeezing of cells resulting from the increased fragility of the tumor nuclei, and the loss of cellular binding material with resulting increased dissociation of tumor cells and the appearance of so-called microadenomas in which there is a pseudoacinar arrangement of nuclei and disappearance of cellular boundaries.

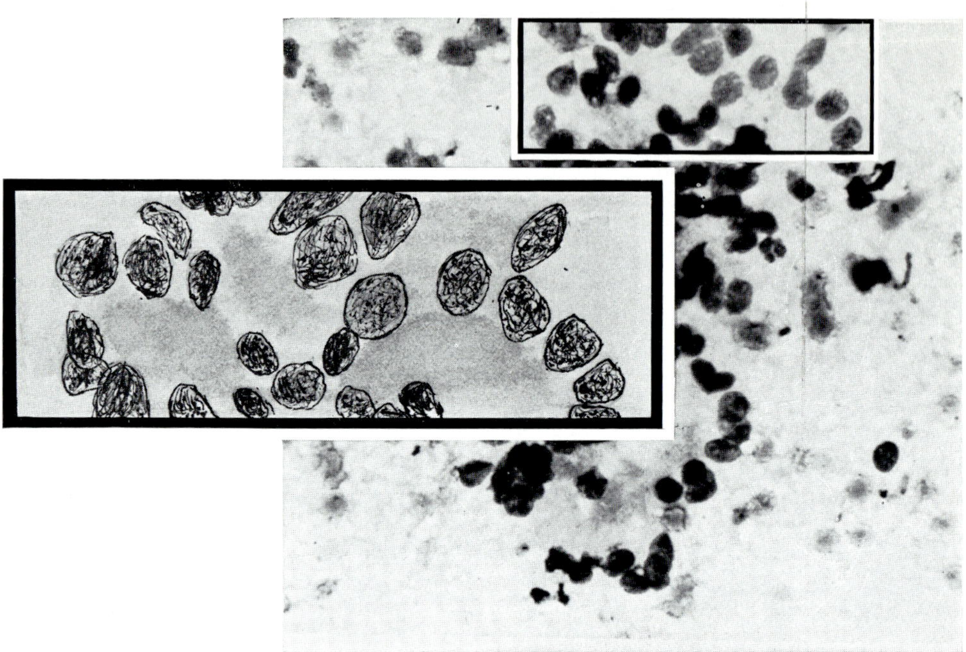

Fig. C.2. — Schematic representation of a well-differentiated carcinoma. The tumor cells have a pseudoacinar arrangement, are without recognizable cell boundaries, and form so-called microadenomas. Such acinar formation is mostly multiple and is seen throughout the entire smear.

Frequently the loss of the sheetlike pattern and the dissociation of cells can be easily seen with low-power magnification. But to make certain of the diagnosis, the other cellular changes must also be taken into account.

The treatment of prostatic carcinoma is conditioned by the spread of the tumor and its grade of malignancy. We know from a great number of statistical studies that well-differentiated adenocarcinomas have a much better prognosis than completely undifferentiated carcinomas. Well-differentiated carcinomas frequently respond to estrogen therapy, often with smaller doses of estrogen used than for less well-differentiated tumors, in which primary estrogen failures are common or only an insufficient cytostatic effect is obtained. In cases of poorly differentiated or even anaplastic tumors, it is best to start radiation therapy as soon as it is established that they do not respond to estrogen.

The cytologic picture — like the histologic — often shows both well-differentiated and less well-differentiated parts in the same tumor. In such cases, therapy is directed to the least differentiated part, even if this is discovered only in a small area.

24

A well-differentiated prostatic carcinoma shows partial preservation of its sheetlike pattern and there are relatively few detached cells. Pathologic nucleoli are infrequent. As has been mentioned already, so-called microadenomas are present. These are nuclei of tumor cells that are arranged in pseudoacinar fashion and lie in a mass of cytoplasm having no recognizable cell boundaries (Fig. C.2).

Moderately well-differentiated carcinomas have marked polymorphism and polychromasia, advanced dissociation of the cell sheets, and numerous isolated tumor cell nuclei or small masses of tumor cells. Large, prominent nucleoli are quite regularly present (Fig. C.3).

Poorly differentiated and undifferentiated prostatic carcinomas are often impressive because of their cellular richness, which frequently causes thick overlapping of cells in

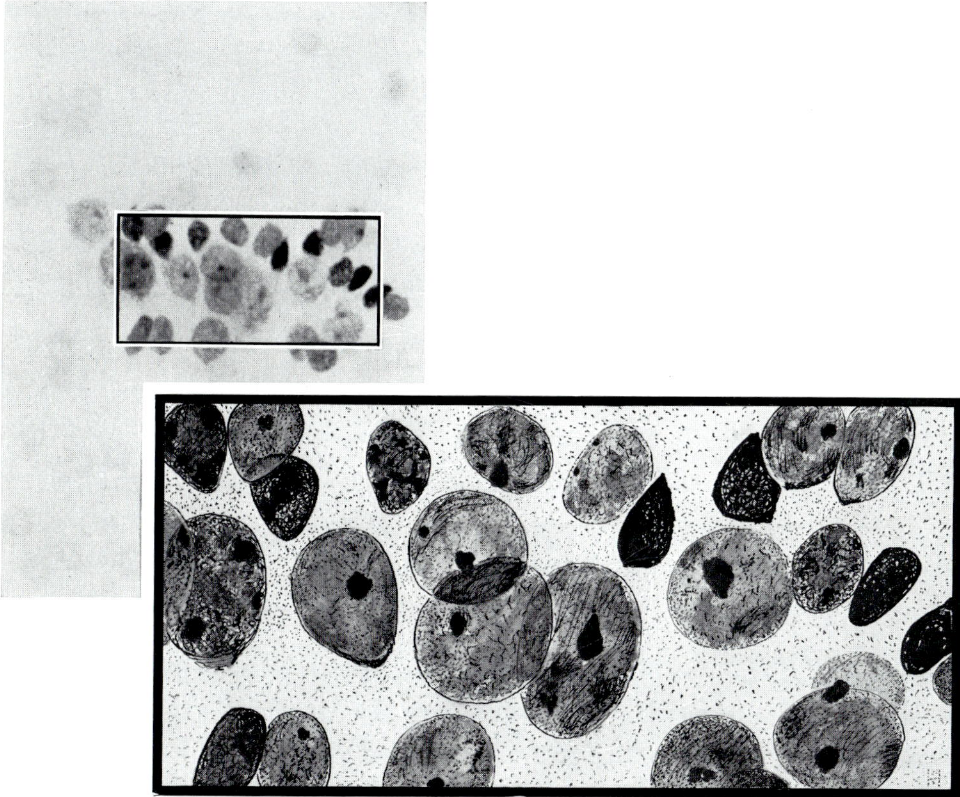

Fig. C.3. — Schematic representation of a moderately well-differentiated prostatic carcinoma. There is a distinct loss of the sheet pattern. Detached aggregates of cells show marked polymorphism and polychromasia, and there are large pathologic nucleoli.

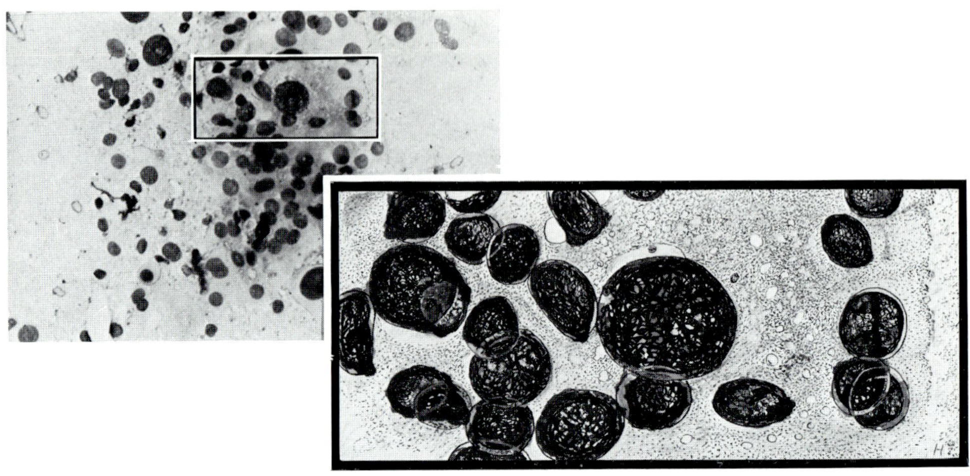

Fig. C.4. – Schematic picture of a poorly differentiated carcinoma. Complete dissociation of tumor nuclei with marked polymorphism and polychromasia.

the smears of aspirated material. The cellular picture appears somewhat monotonous. Sheets of adherent cells are no longer recognizable, the nuclei are polymorphic and polychromatic, and most have no cytoplasm. Cellular dissociation is widespread and throughout the smear a sheet pattern is lacking. Large nucleoli are common and may predominate (Fig. C.4).

Because of increased fragility the tumor nuclei often appear to be squashed.

4. Therapy-Dependent Effects

Following orchiectomy, atrophy of prostatic epithelium often develops due to widespread stimulating effects of the androgens on both the prostate and the carcinoma. Cytologically, except for polymorphism, the atrophic cells show no remarkable changes.

In conservative treatment of prostatic carcinoma, contrasexual hormones are used, most often estrogens in various stored forms or synthetic preparations with an estrogen-like action (e. g., stilbene). Cases so treated show massive squamous cell metaplasia in the cytologic preparation. These cells are non-keratinized, rich in glycogen, and usually referred to as "glycogenic cells" (Fig. C.5). They arise from hyperplasia of the estrogen-stimulated basal cell layer of normal glandular epithelium. The carcinoma cells themselves, according to all observers, show no squamous metaplasia. However,

26

slight hydropic swelling of carcinoma cells may confuse the inexperienced observer. Since nearly 80% of carcinomas are treated first with hormones, all changes in the nuclei of tumor cells must be carefully evaluated. These nuclear changes are already apparent after 3–4 weeks (100–400 mg estrogen) and consist of distinct netlike loosening of the nucleoplasm with disruption and vacuolation of the interior of the nucleus. In later stages there is pyknosis, karyolysis, and increased mucin production. In a well-treated carcinoma, only a few or perhaps no tumor cells will be discovered in the biopsy.

Most squamous epithelium concurrently aspirated comes not from carcinomatous tissue but from the metaplastic normal glandular tissue of adjacent structures. According to current ideas of hormone action, contrasexual therapy with estrogens or substances with a hormone-like action has a direct effect on the tumor cells and especially

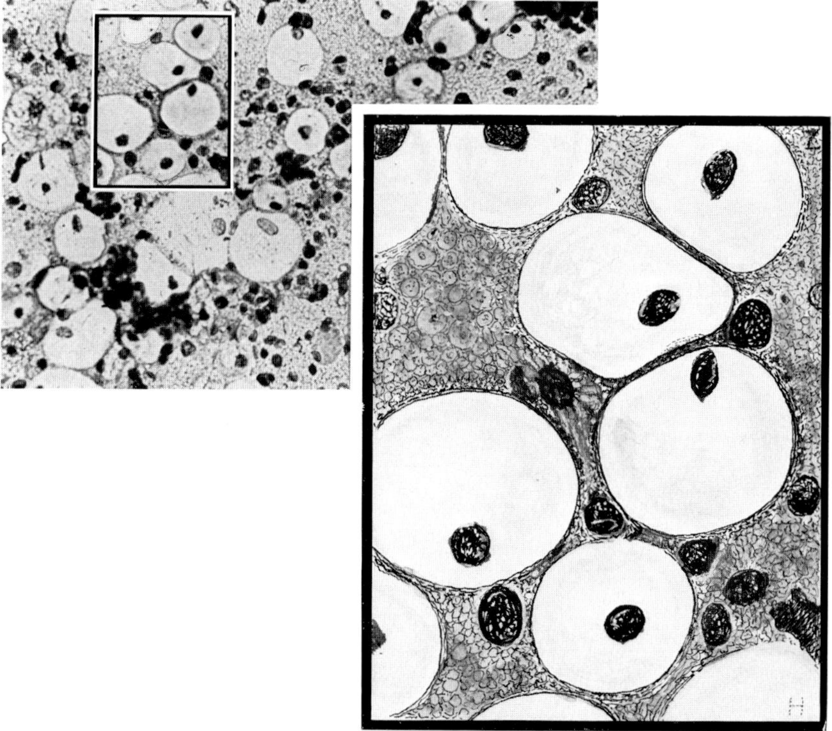

Fig. C. 5. — Schematic picture of estrogen-induced squamous epithelial metaplasia in nodular hyperplasia of the prostate (adenoma). Superficial cells like the metaplastic ones are rich in glycogen. They arise under estrogen stimulation from hyperplasia of the basal cells of normal glandular epithelium.

on their nuclei. With antiandrogens (e. g., cyproterone acetate), the androgen receptors are blocked by competitive arrest at the receptor organ (prostatic epithelium). Experimentally, after similar periods of time the degenerative changes in tumor cells known to occur after either androgen or estrogen treatments cannot be distinguished. Squamous epithelial metaplasia is less with antiandrogen therapy.

Hormone-resistant carcinomas that are inoperable are treated with radiation. Following cobalt radiation (6000 r), cytological smears contain large giant cells showing partially coalesced nucleoplasm and nuclear vacuolation. There are sporadic cells showing pyknosis and karyolysis; changes that can be interpreted as neither an undifferentiated nor a highly malignant tumor. Tumor cells that do not show such changes must be regarded either as persistent carcinoma that escaped destruction by the radiation or as a recurrence.

5. Cells Concomitantly Aspirated from Neighboring Organs

Even with the best technique of transrectal aspiration biopsy, cells from neighboring organs are sometimes included in the smears of the biopsy lying alongside the sheets of adherent prostatic cells and may be a source of diagnostic error. For the most part such cells are found in one smear only. The first tissue to be penetrated during the puncture is of course the rectal mucosa. This is particularly likely to happen when the needle is withdrawn from the prostate. Rectal epithelium may often be dragged along if the pressure in the syringe has not been equalized by freeing the plunger.

Rectal cells have a large, oval-shaped nucleus and abundant cytoplasm that often has a granular appearance. They show none of the signs of malignancy. Typical goblet cells are seldom seen. Frequently rectal contents and masses of bacteria are also aspirated.

If the biopsy needle penetrates too deeply, bladder epithelium and urine may be aspirated. Because of osmotic cytolysis, the prostatic cells may then become indistinct and difficult to interpret. In addition, such smears are either cloudy or contain more or less typical urine crystals.

Transitional epithelium from the bladder is usually arranged in sheets and is recognized by the large, round, somewhat plump nuclei and abundant cytoplasm that stains blue with the May-Grünwald-Giemsa stain.

Spermatozoa are sometimes difficult to recognize because they may become altered by cytolysis and have no recognizable tails. They may be aspirated from the prostatic urethra, but they come mostly from the ampulla.

28

Epithelium from the seminal vesicles is most difficult to interpret. As well as very pronounced polymorphism, there is also marked dissociation of cells. Numerous nucleoli are present also because of the high functional differentiation of the epithelium, but they have no malignant significance. The cytoplasm is abundant and commonly shows small or large vacuoles, sporadic yellow granules, and small nuclear fragments resembling phagocytosed spermatozoa heads. However, the frequent finding of whole sperm in the neighborhood of these cells and the appearance of streaming make the diagnosis easier. There are no malignant characteristics.

D. Diagnostic Cytology

1. Nodular Hyperplasia (Adenoma) of the Prostate

Fig. D.1. – On the *left* is the histologic preparation, showing nodular hyperplasia of the prostate (HE, 250×). The glands and muscle have a regular arrangement and the epithelial cells lining the glands are uniform and form papillae within the lumens. The muscle fibers are clearly seen between the glands. On the *right* is a cytologic preparation from the same patient (May-Grünwald-Giemsa, 250×). Notice the sharp differentiation of the cell nuclei. The epithelial cells are layered in sheets, whereas in the histologic preparation they form glands.

Fig. D.2. – Sheet of prostatic epithelial cells with nearly uniform, round nuclei typical of nodular hyperplasia of the prostate (adenomyosis, May-Grünwald-Giemsa, 400×).

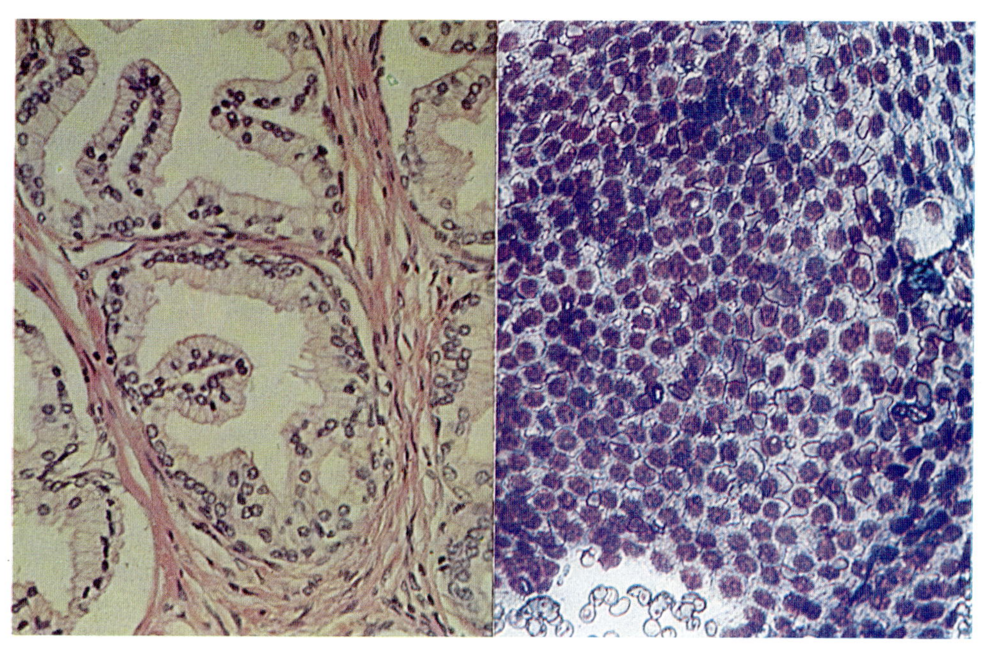

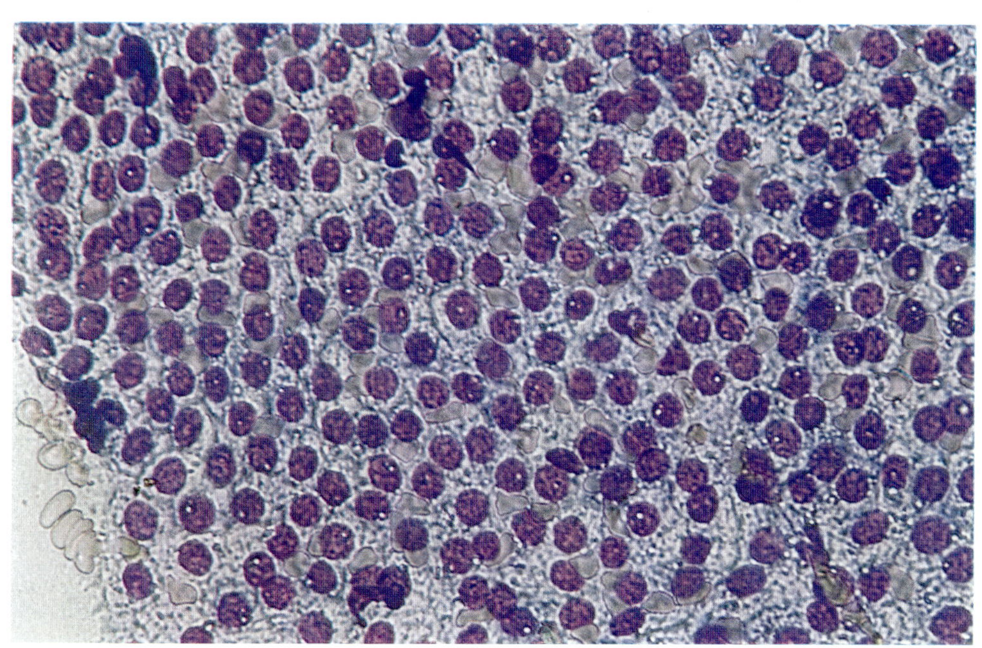

Fig. D.3. — Multiple sheets of prostatic epithelium lying side by side. Above the middle of the picture the cells overlap each other in an irregular fashion, forming a double layer. There are almost no detached single cells (May-Grünwald-Giemsa, 250×).

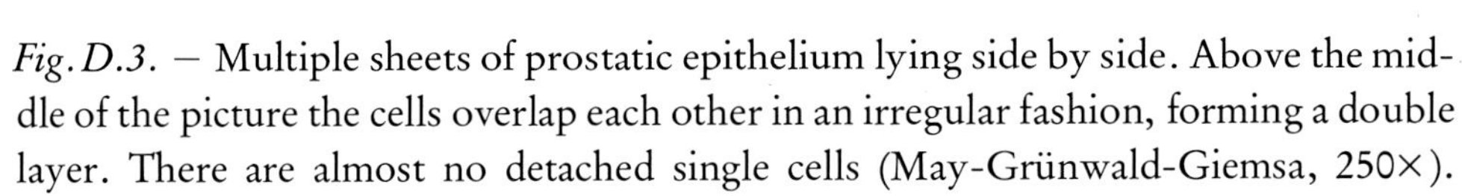

Fig. D.4. — Sheet of normal prostatic epithelium overlaid with diffusely distributed granules. This is seen only in normal glands. Their composition and importance are as yet unknown. There are also aggregates of simultaneously aspirated erythrocytes in the field (May-Grünwald-Giemsa, 400×).

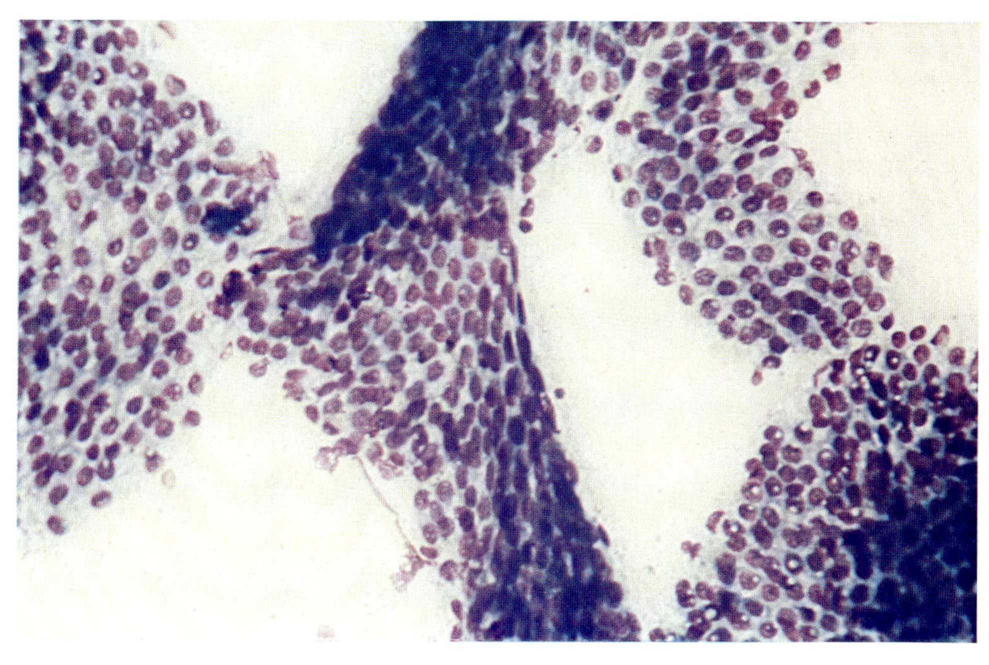

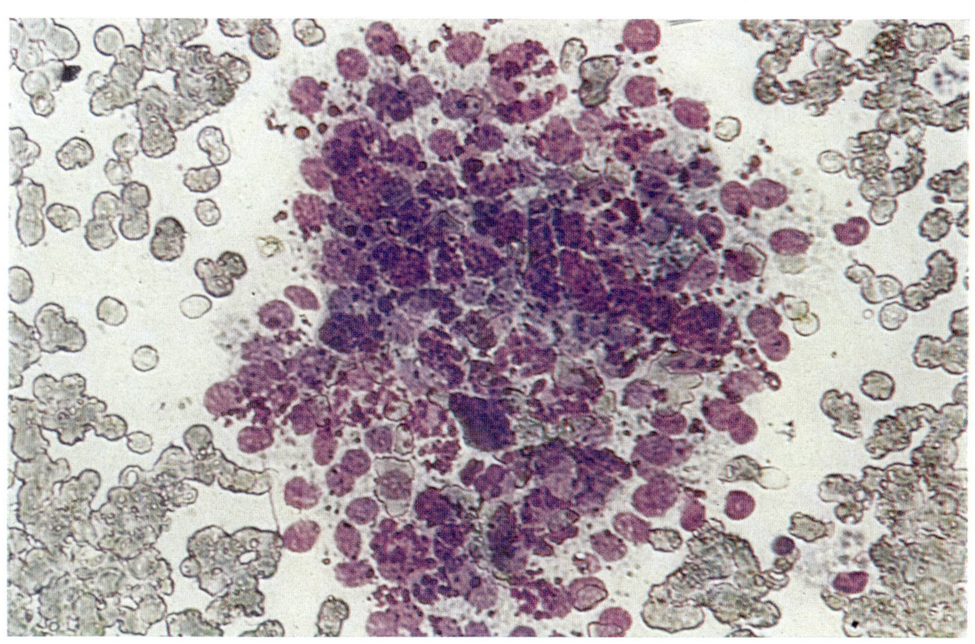

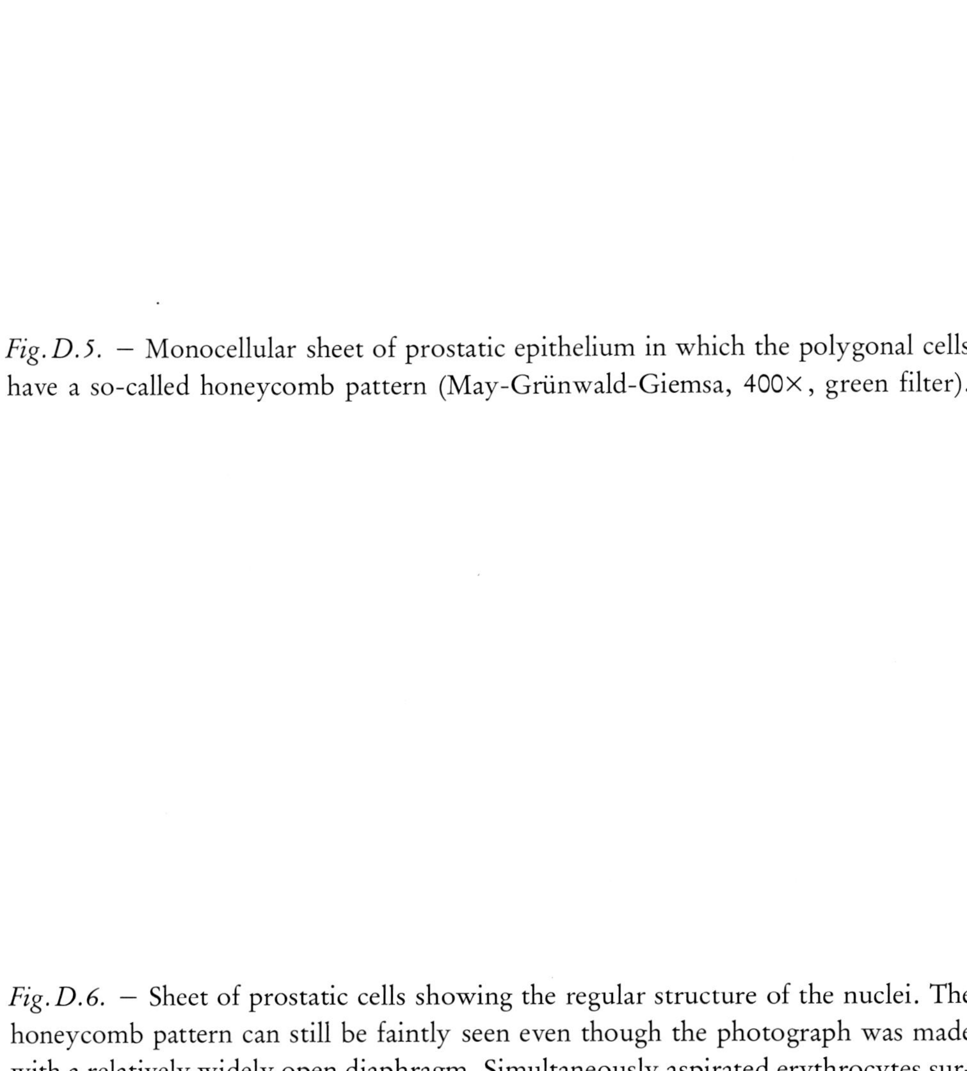

Fig. D.5. – Monocellular sheet of prostatic epithelium in which the polygonal cells have a so-called honeycomb pattern (May-Grünwald-Giemsa, 400×, green filter).

Fig. D.6. – Sheet of prostatic cells showing the regular structure of the nuclei. The honeycomb pattern can still be faintly seen even though the photograph was made with a relatively widely open diaphragm. Simultaneously aspirated erythrocytes surround the sheet of cells (May-Grünwald-Giemsa, 400×).

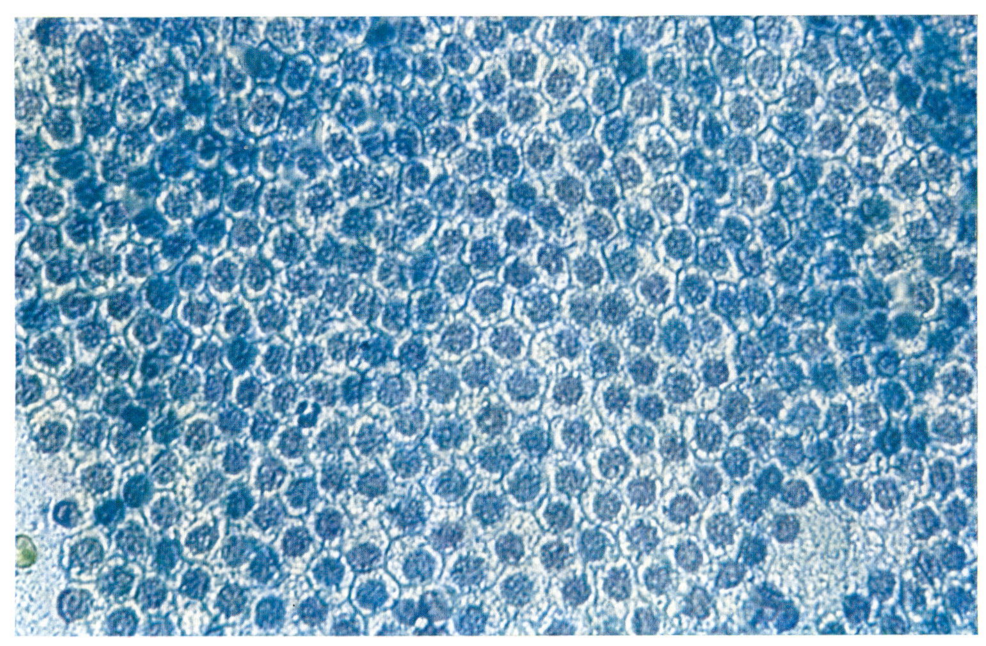

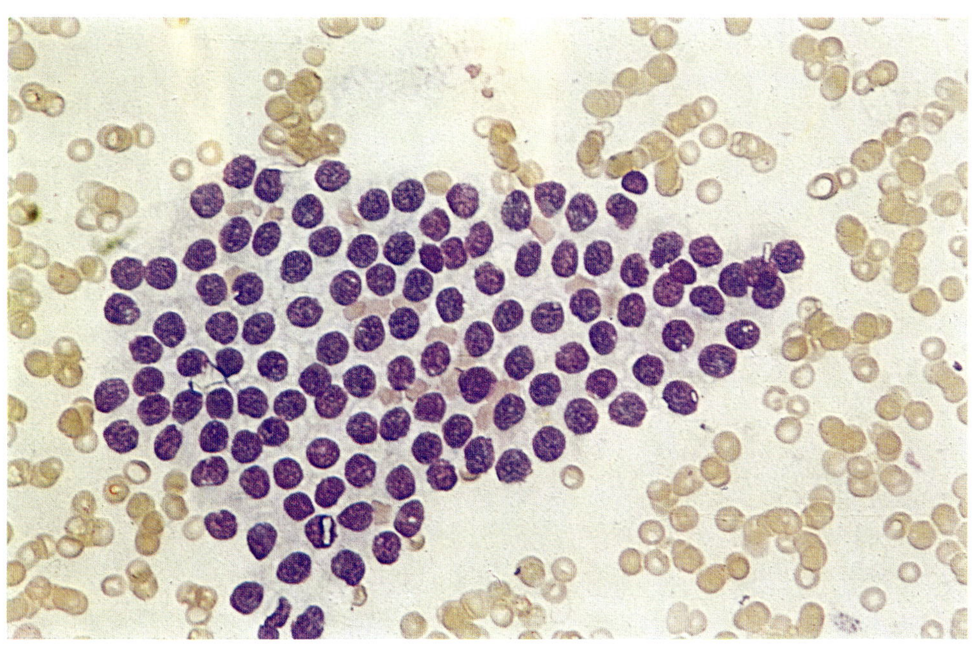

Fig. D.7. – Monocellular sheet of prostatic epithelium in which detached cells overlap. The nuclear polymorphism is within normal limits. The internal structure of the cells appears to be regular. The solitary, small vacuoles probably are caused by the air drying. The cytoplasm is partly overlaid by bluish granules (May-Grünwald-Giemsa, 400×).

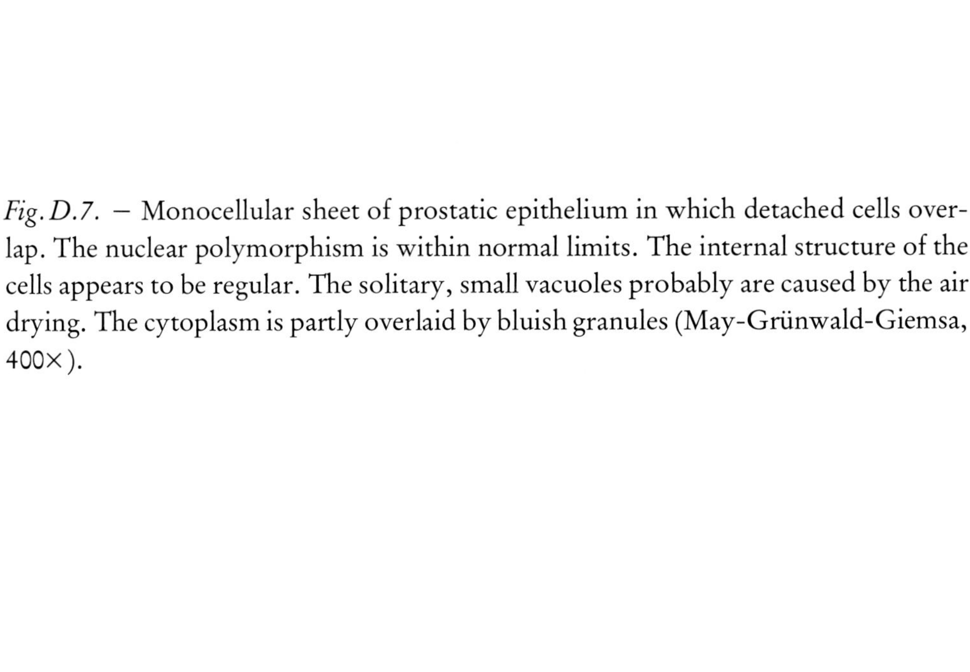

Fig. D.8. – Sheet of prostatic cells in which the honeycomb pattern is made especially clear by completely closing the diaphragm (May-Grünwald-Giemsa, 400×).

36

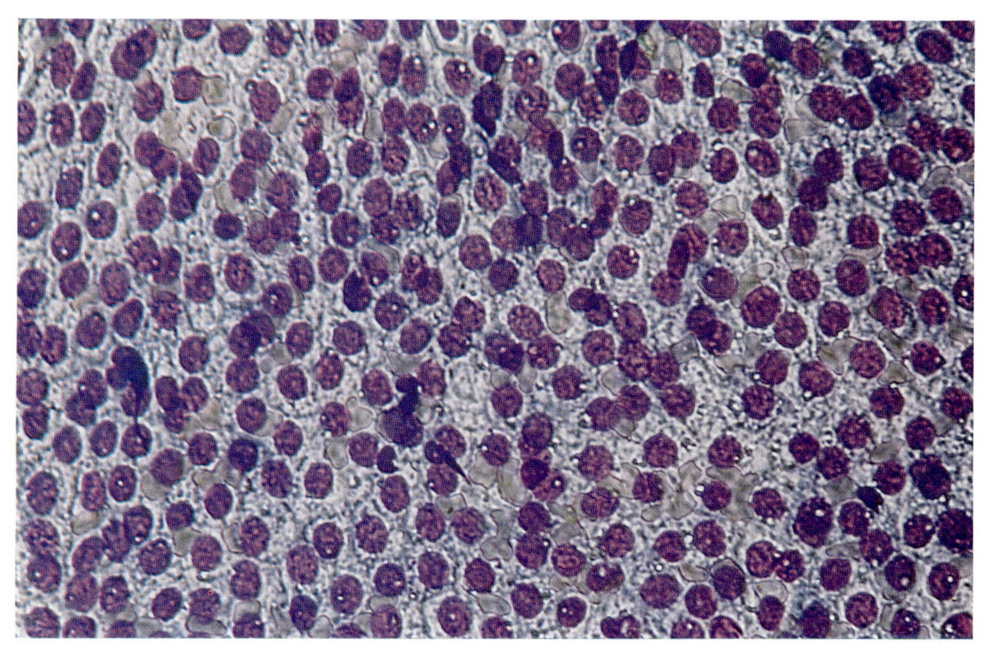

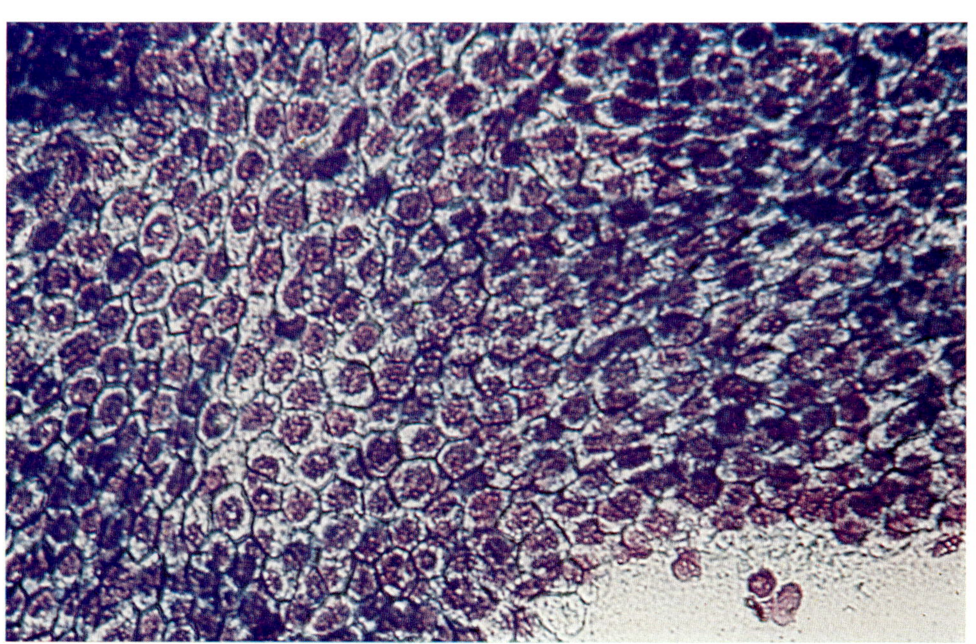

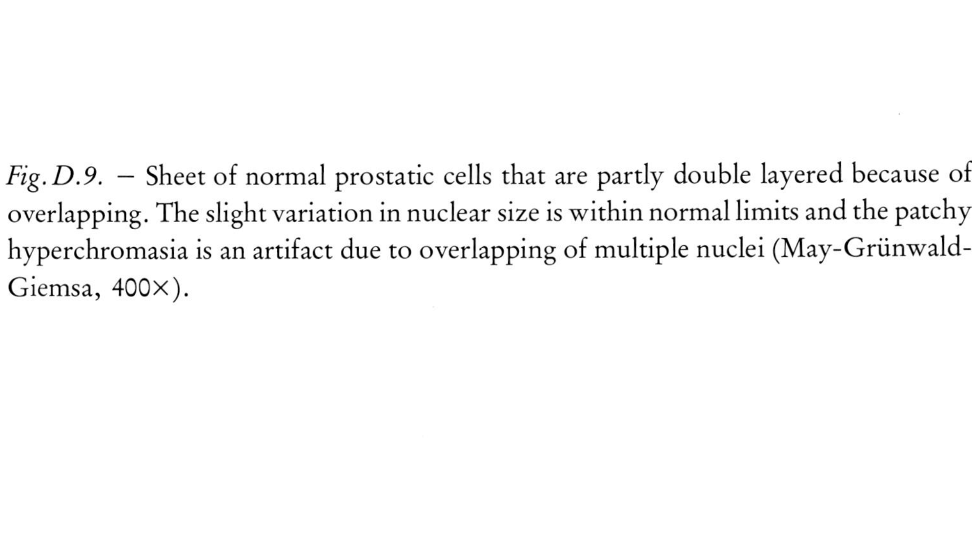

Fig. D.9. — Sheet of normal prostatic cells that are partly double layered because of overlapping. The slight variation in nuclear size is within normal limits and the patchy hyperchromasia is an artifact due to overlapping of multiple nuclei (May-Grünwald-Giemsa, 400×).

Fig. D.10. — Sheet of prostatic cells with multilayered nuclei in the upper right-hand corner. The overlapping is most likely due in part to the smearing, but it may also be due to distortion of the glands (May-Grünwald-Giemsa, 400×).

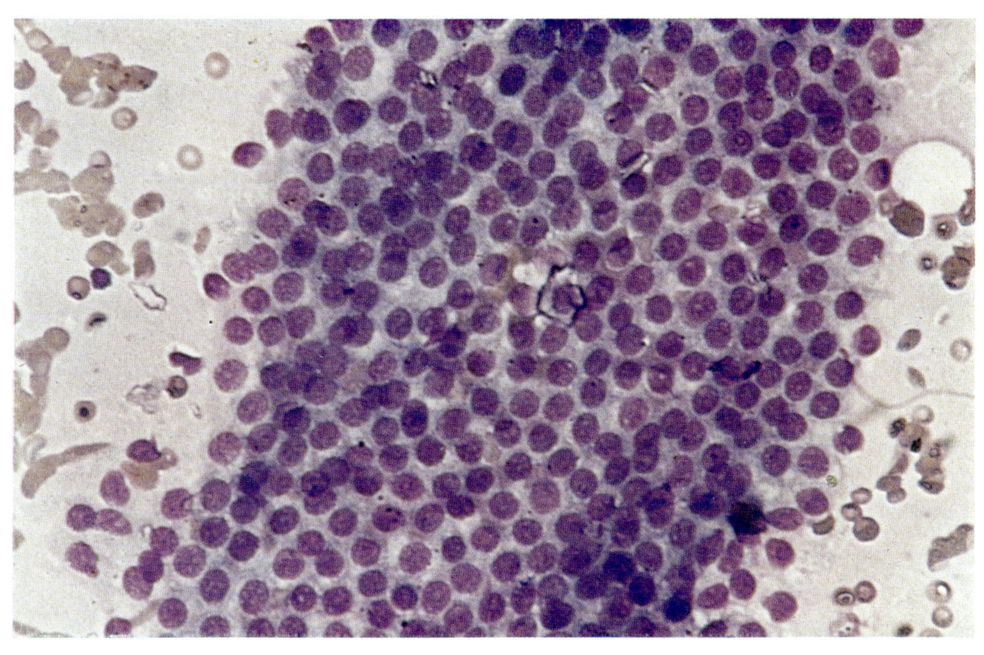

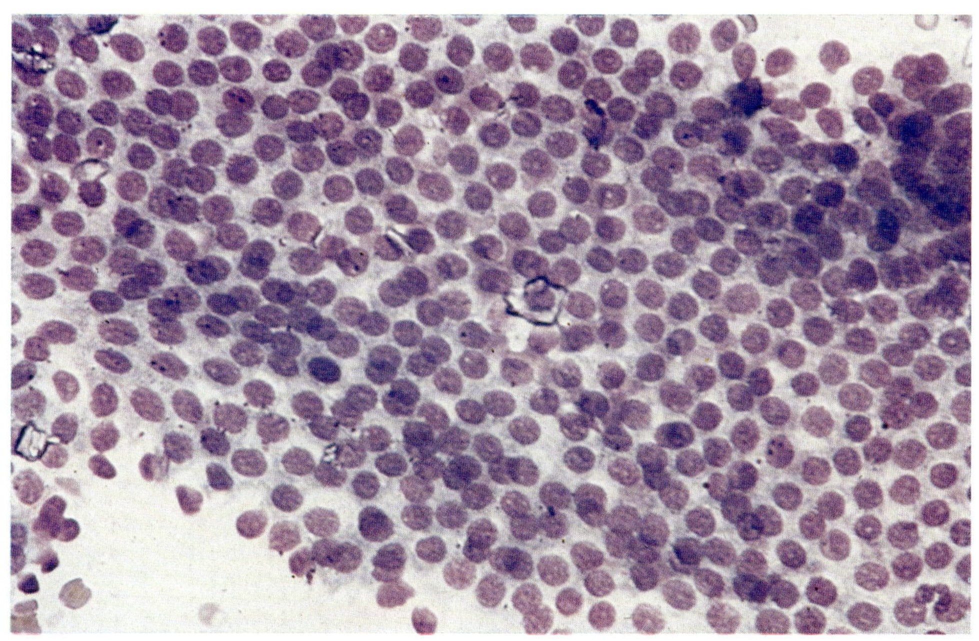

39

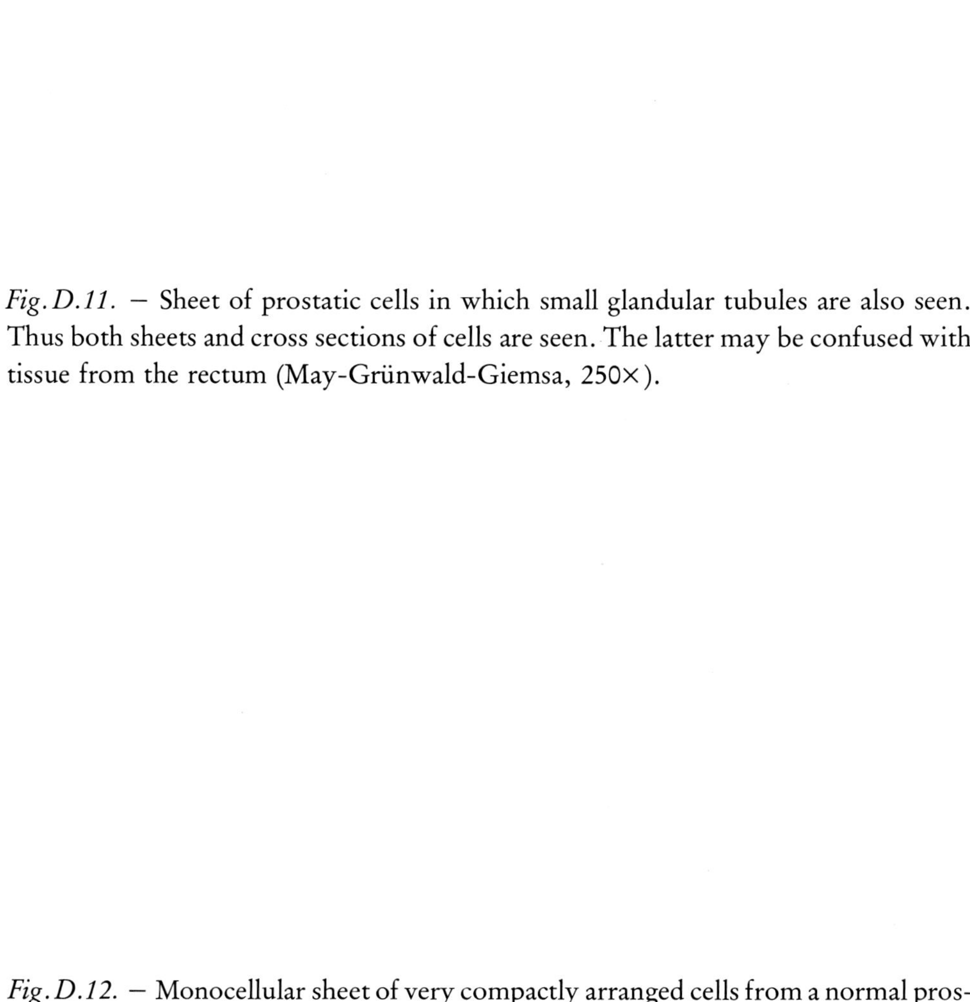

Fig. D.11. − Sheet of prostatic cells in which small glandular tubules are also seen. Thus both sheets and cross sections of cells are seen. The latter may be confused with tissue from the rectum (May-Grünwald-Giemsa, 250×).

Fig. D.12. − Monocellular sheet of very compactly arranged cells from a normal prostate. The cell borders are clearly seen. The somewhat bizarre, polymorphic nuclei in the lower left-hand corner of the illustration are due partly to overlapping and partly to imperfect smearing (HE, 400×).

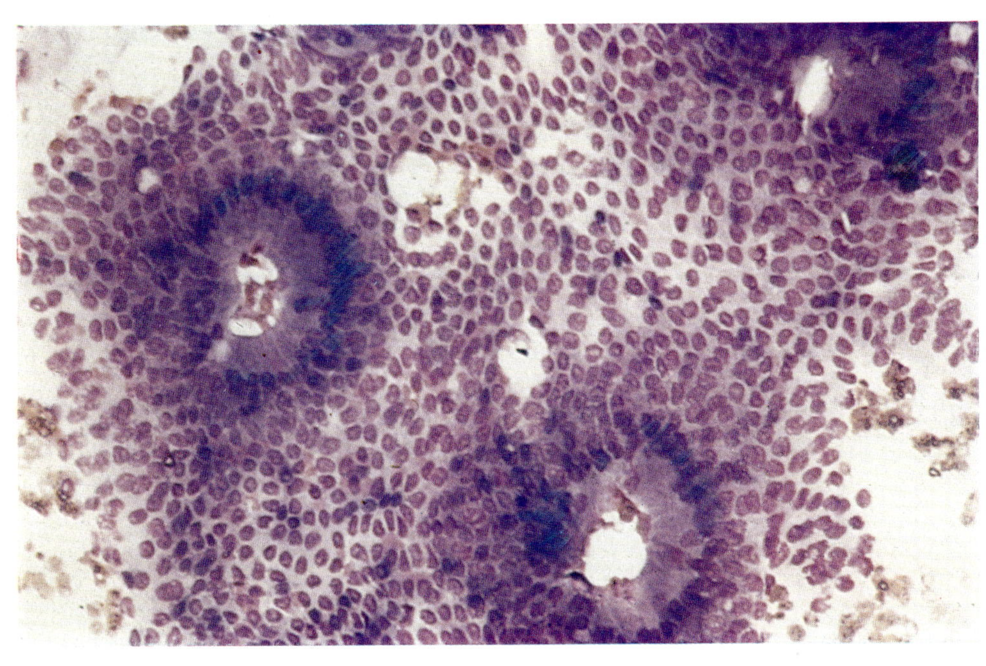

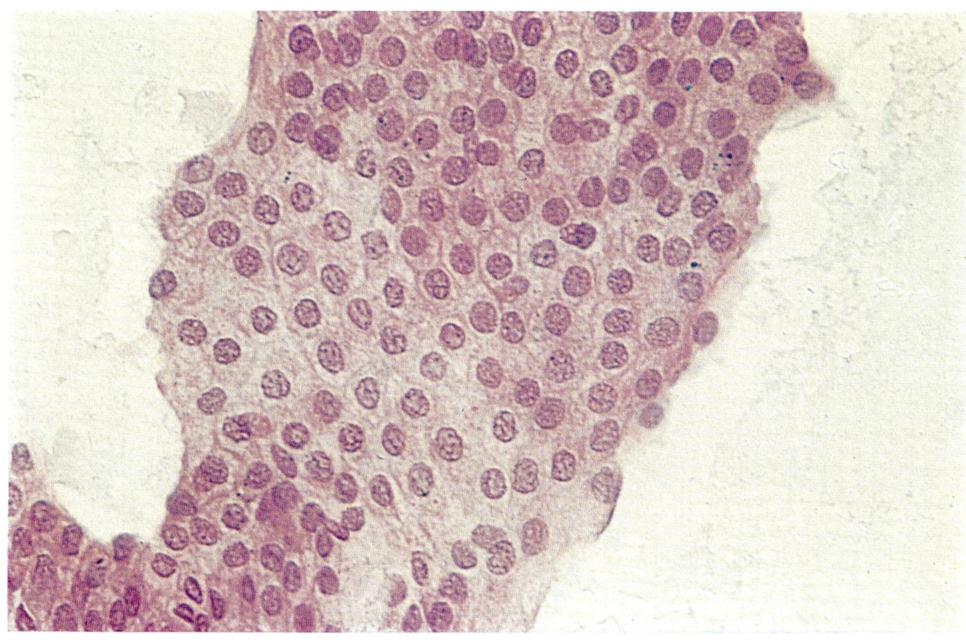

Fig. D.13. – Sheet of prostatic cells in which overlapping due to squirting the aspirated material onto the slide has caused an irregular appearance. However there are no characteristics of malignancy (May-Grünwald-Giemsa, 250×).

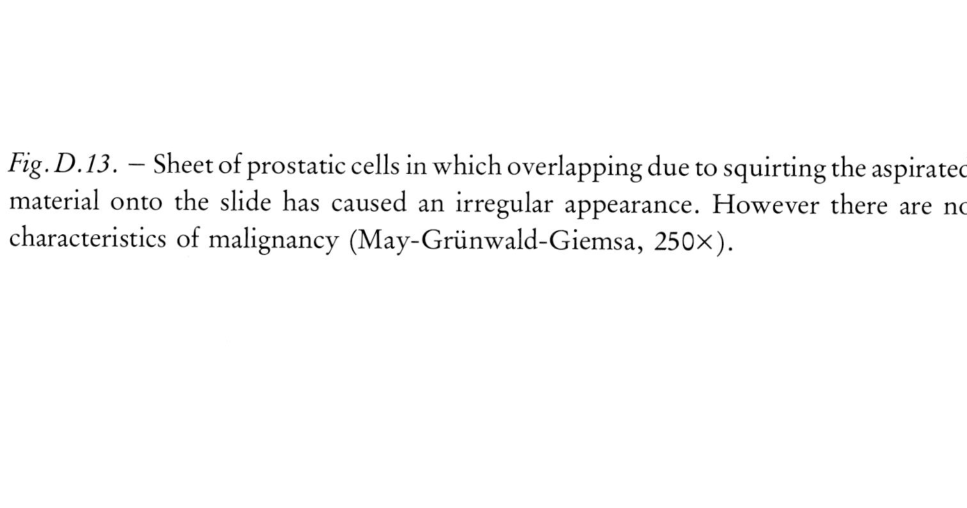

Fig. D.14. – Prostatic smear in which the sheet seems to have been unrolled from both sides. This appearance results from ejection from the canula (May-Grünwald-Giemsa, 250×).

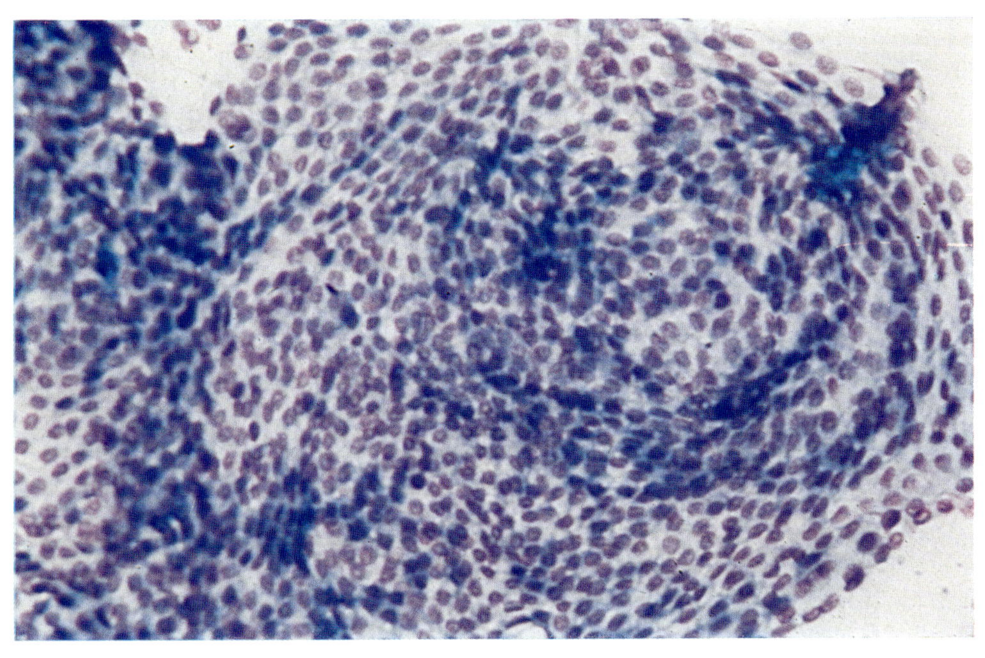

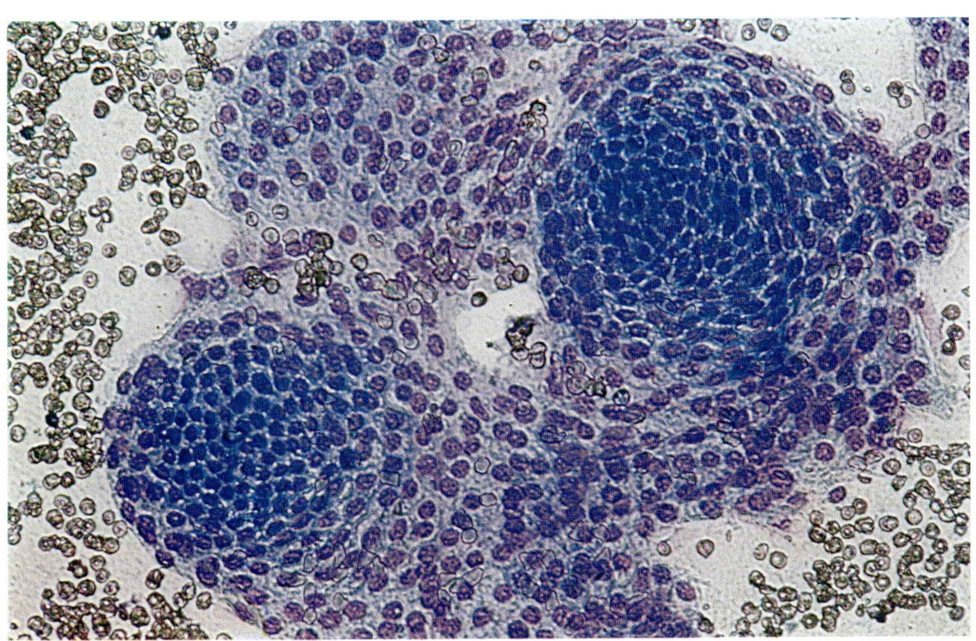

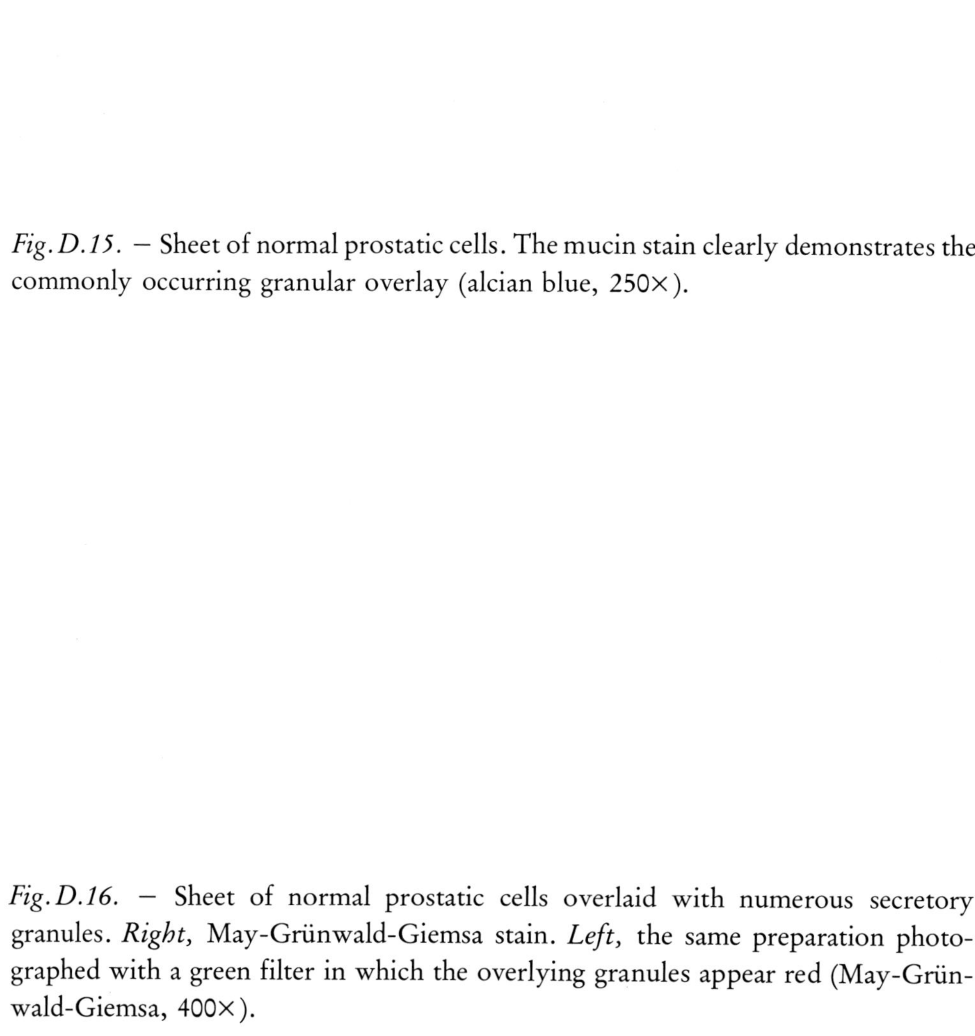

Fig.D.15. — Sheet of normal prostatic cells. The mucin stain clearly demonstrates the commonly occurring granular overlay (alcian blue, 250×).

Fig.D.16. — Sheet of normal prostatic cells overlaid with numerous secretory granules. *Right,* May-Grünwald-Giemsa stain. *Left,* the same preparation photographed with a green filter in which the overlying granules appear red (May-Grünwald-Giemsa, 400×).

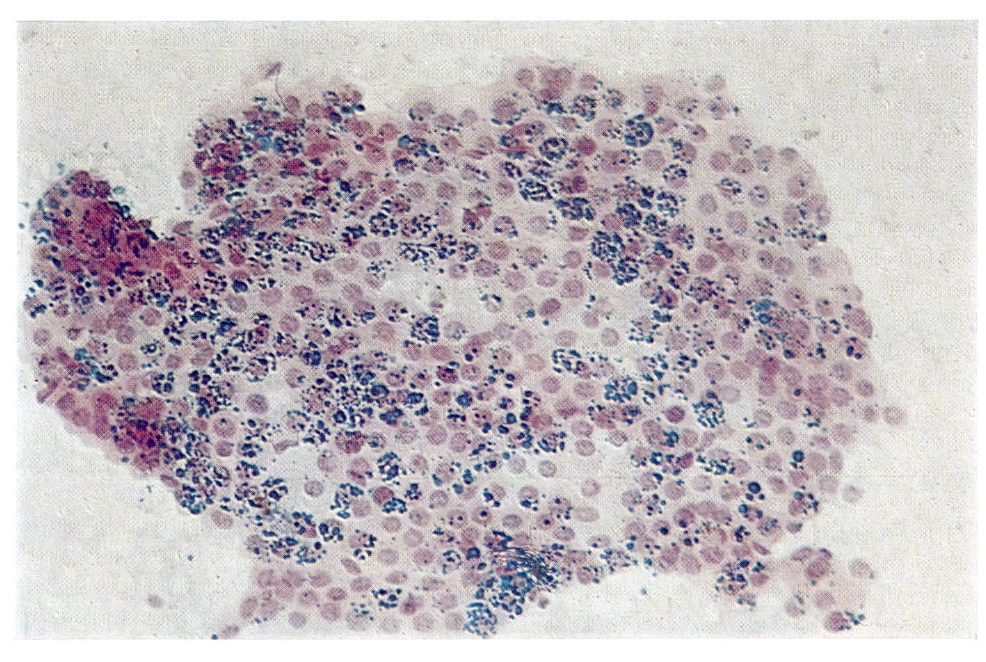

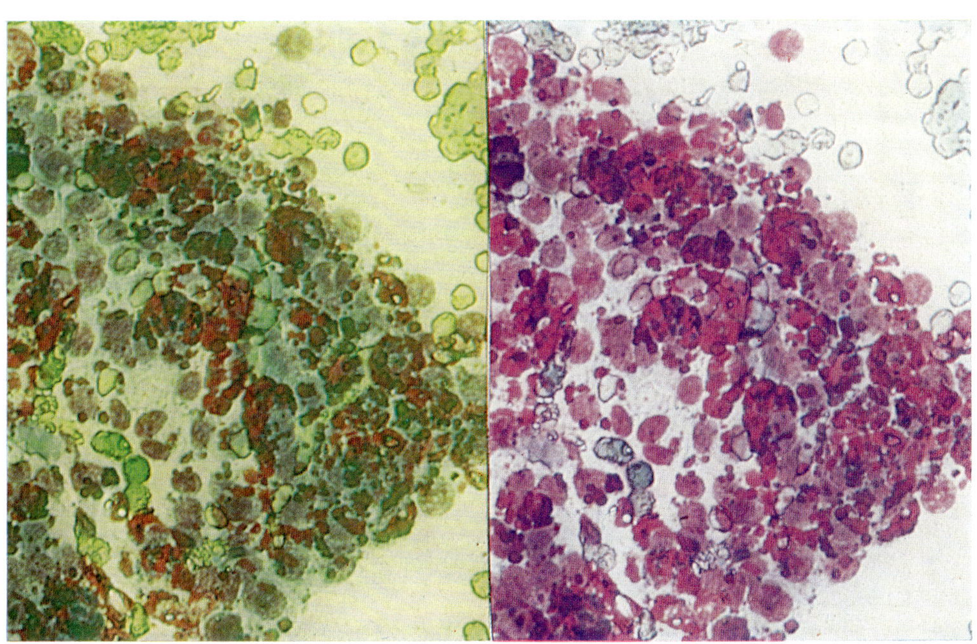

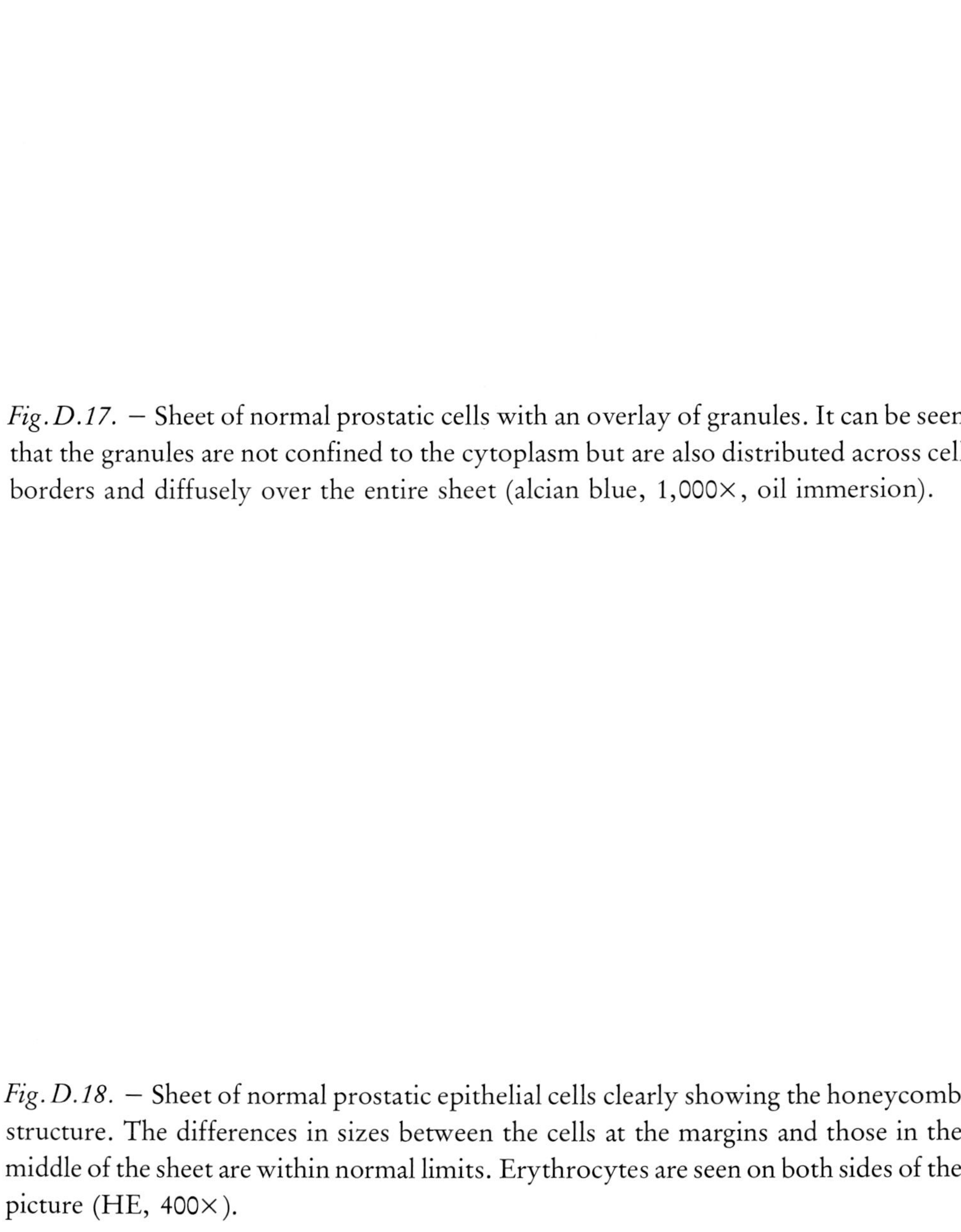

Fig. D.17. – Sheet of normal prostatic cells with an overlay of granules. It can be seen that the granules are not confined to the cytoplasm but are also distributed across cell borders and diffusely over the entire sheet (alcian blue, 1,000×, oil immersion).

Fig. D.18. – Sheet of normal prostatic epithelial cells clearly showing the honeycomb structure. The differences in sizes between the cells at the margins and those in the middle of the sheet are within normal limits. Erythrocytes are seen on both sides of the picture (HE, 400×).

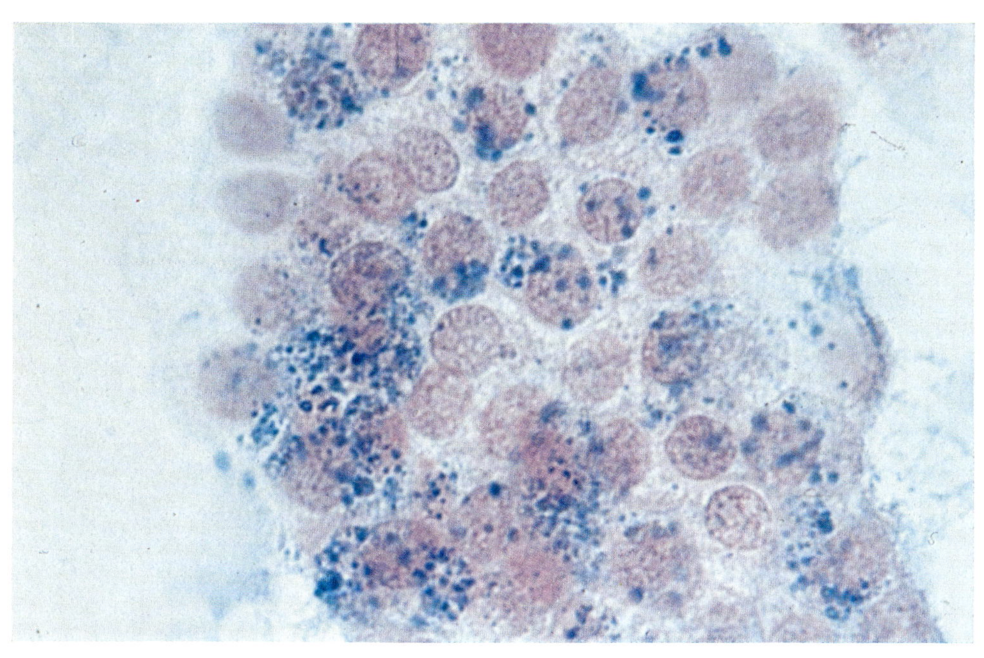

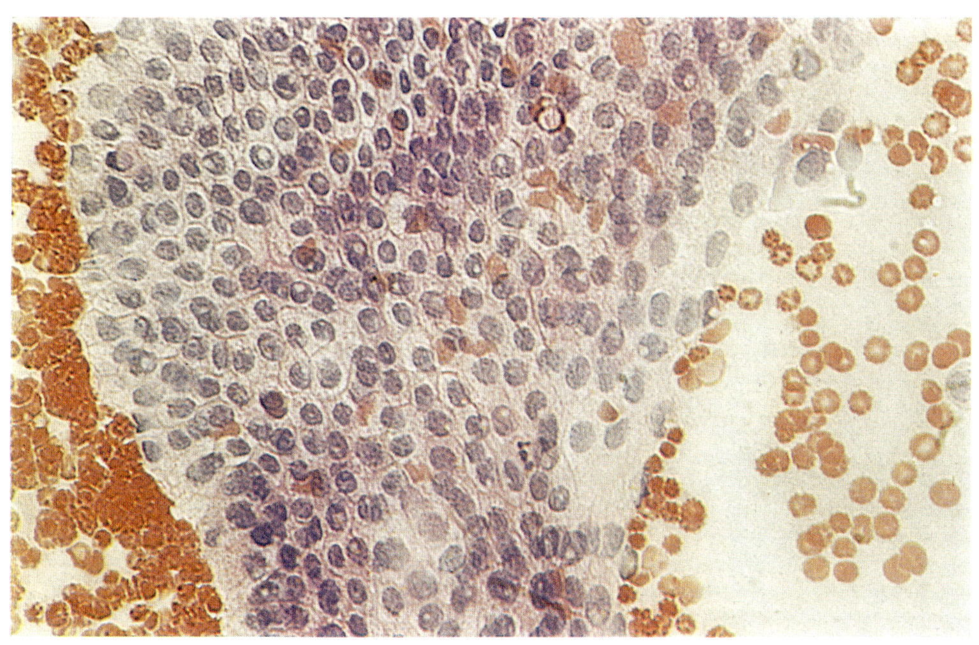

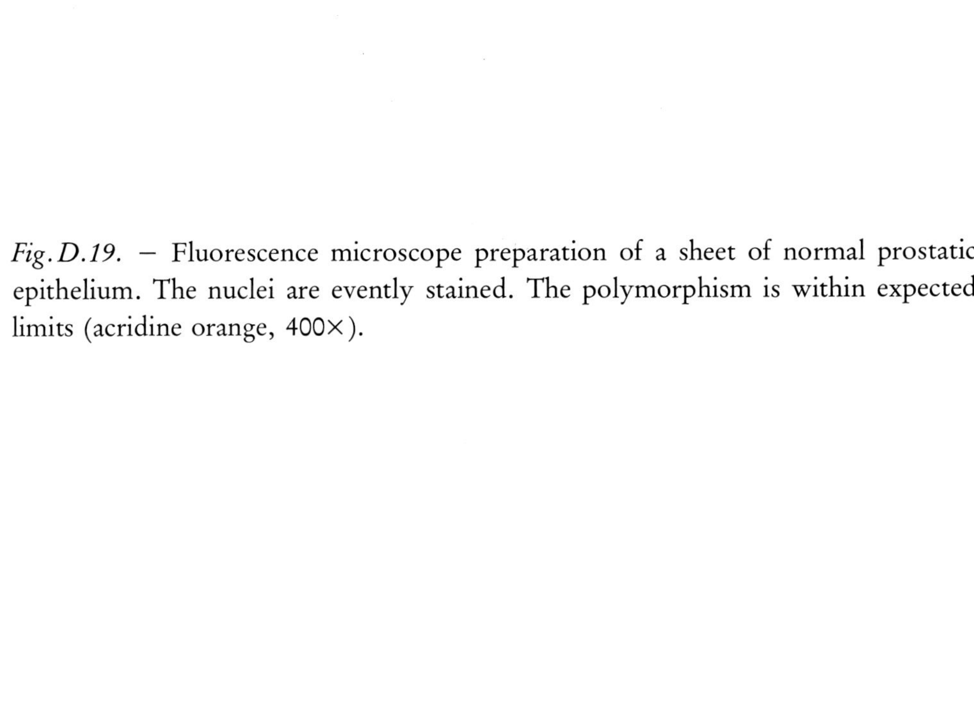

Fig. D.19. – Fluorescence microscope preparation of a sheet of normal prostatic epithelium. The nuclei are evenly stained. The polymorphism is within expected limits (acridine orange, 400×).

Fig. D.20. – Sheet of prostatic cells in which overlapping of cells has caused an irregular appearance. Such a finding is caused by the smear technique and is normal (May-Grünwald-Giemsa, 250×).

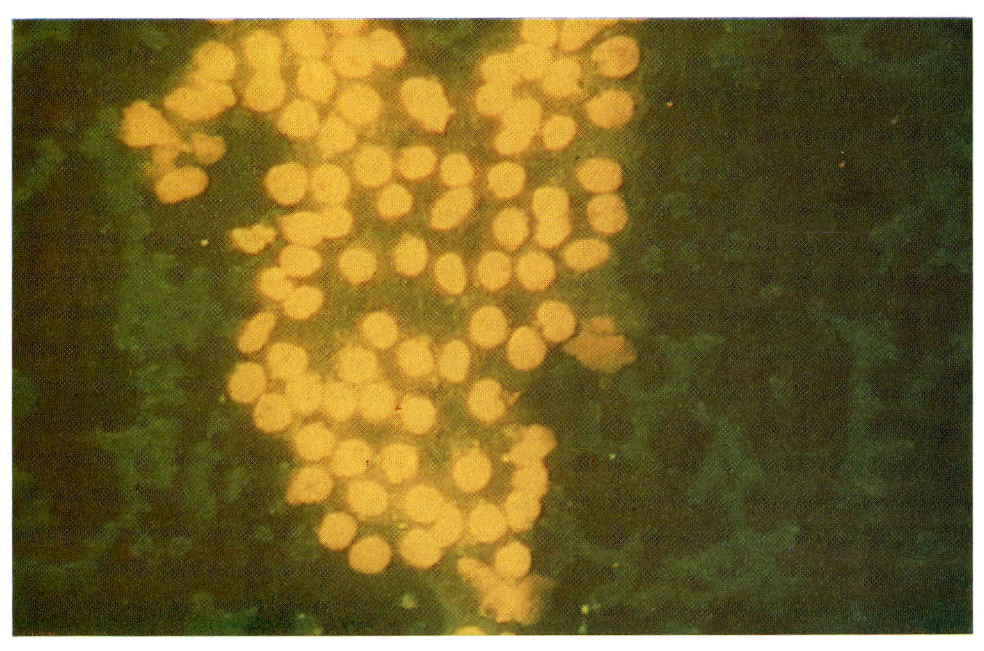

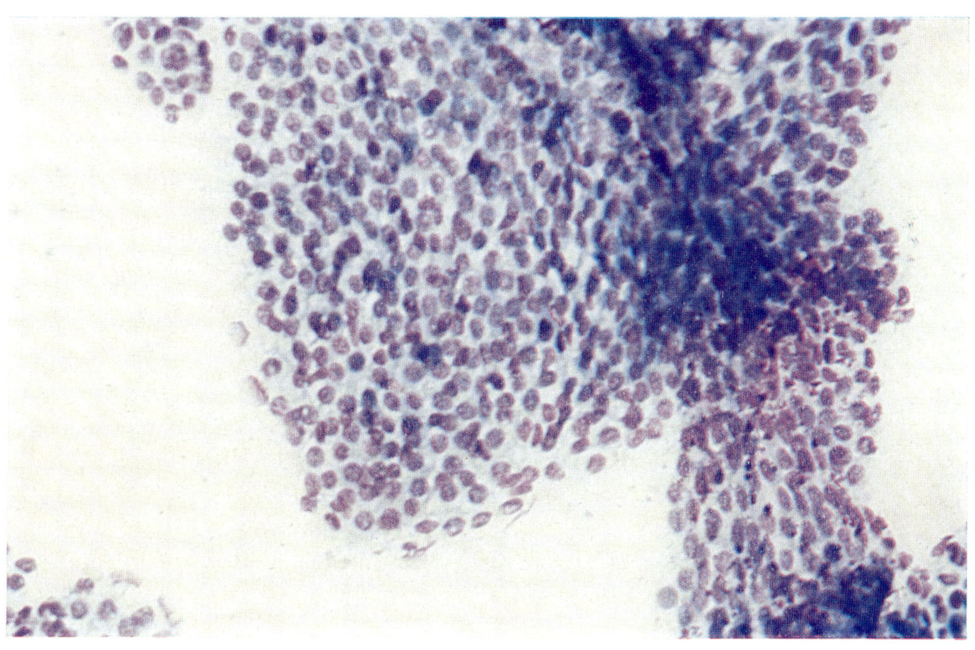

Fig.D.21. – Sheet of normal prostatic cells overlaid by polychromatic, purple-blue secretory granules (May-Grünwald-Giemsa, 400×).

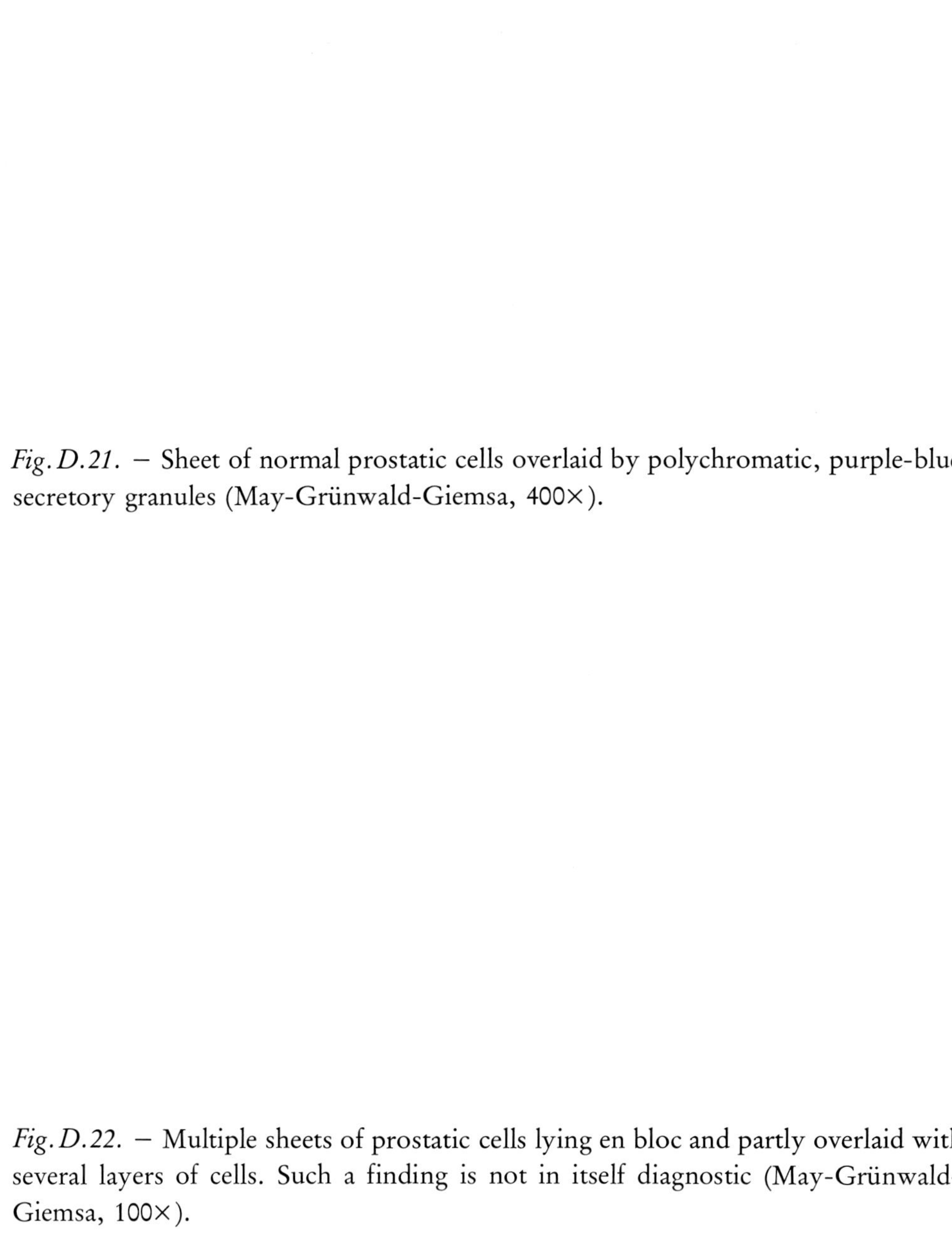

Fig.D.22. – Multiple sheets of prostatic cells lying en bloc and partly overlaid with several layers of cells. Such a finding is not in itself diagnostic (May-Grünwald-Giemsa, 100×).

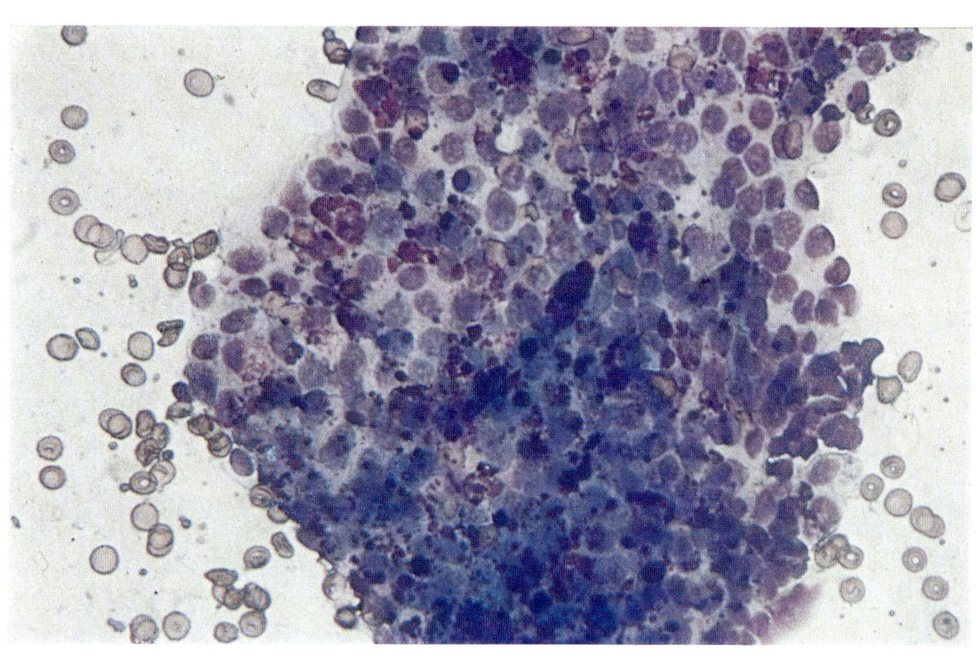

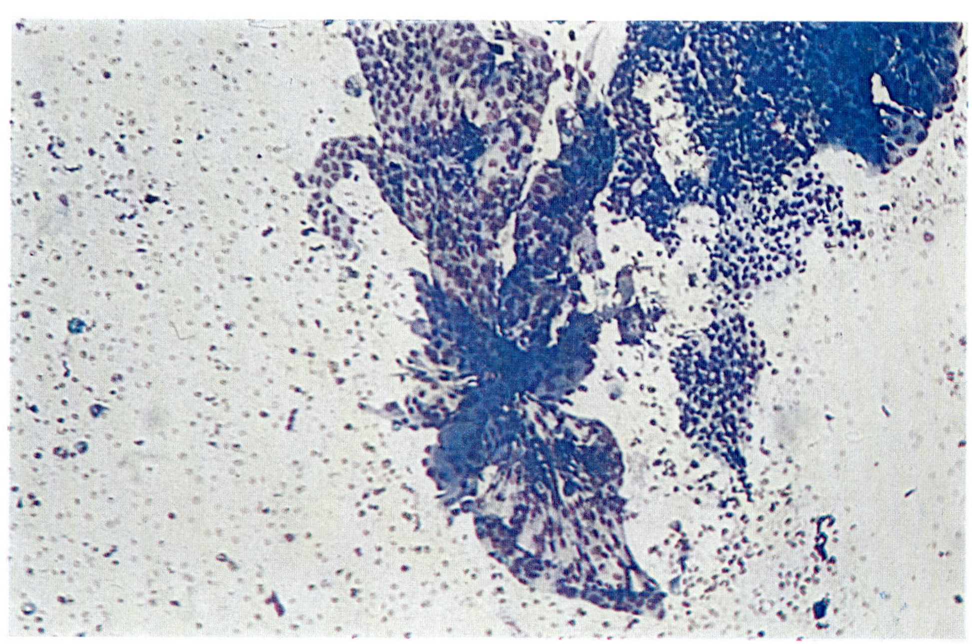

Fig. D.23. – Prostatic cells from a young person (17 years). The rather marked polymorphism of cell nuclei is remarkable. There is likewise little of a honeycomb pattern. The cells lie on top of each other in part and are distributed in many large clumps. There are, however, no malignant characteristics (May-Grünwald-Giemsa, 400×).

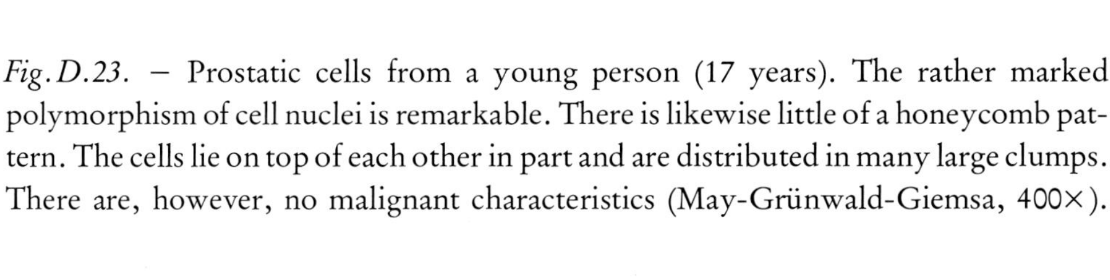

Fig. D.24. – Prostate of a young person. Granular overlay of the sheet of cells on the right. Frequent overlapping and multilayering of epithelial cells (May-Grünwald-Giemsa, 400×).

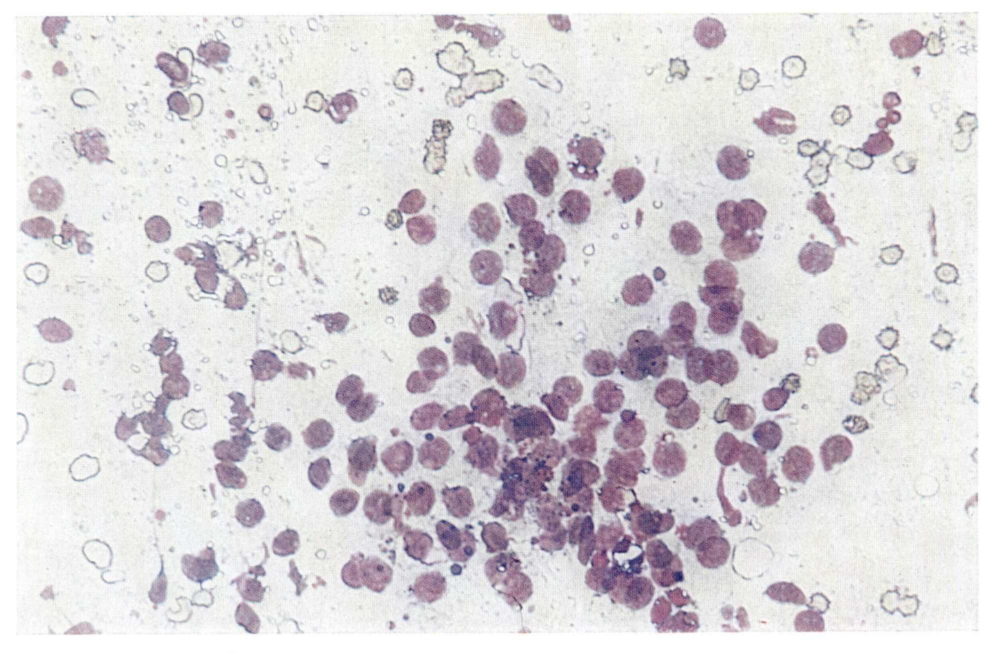

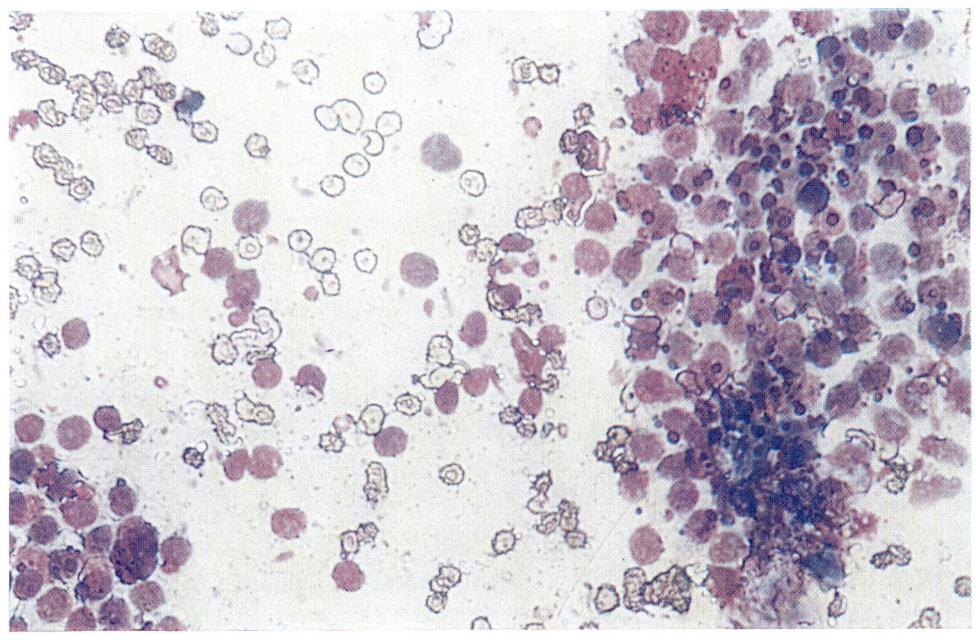

Fig. D.25. — Prostatic cells of a juvenile. The dispersion of cells is quite apparent and the cells show little adhesion and no honeycomb pattern. There is a granular overlay. Detached cells are normal in the young (May-Grünwald-Giemsa, 400×).

2. Prostatitis

a) Acute Prostatitis

Fig. D.26. — Comparison of the histology and cytology of acute prostatitis. On the *left* is the histologic preparation of a harpoon biopsy in which the lumens of the glands contain polymorphonuclear leukocytes and inflammatory fibrinous exudate. There are also a few leukocytes in the stroma (HE, 250×). On the *right* is the aspiration biopsy. The prostatic epithelial cells appear loosened by edema, and the entire sheet of cells is infiltrated and surrounded by polymorphonuclear granulocytes (May-Grünwald-Giemsa, 400×).

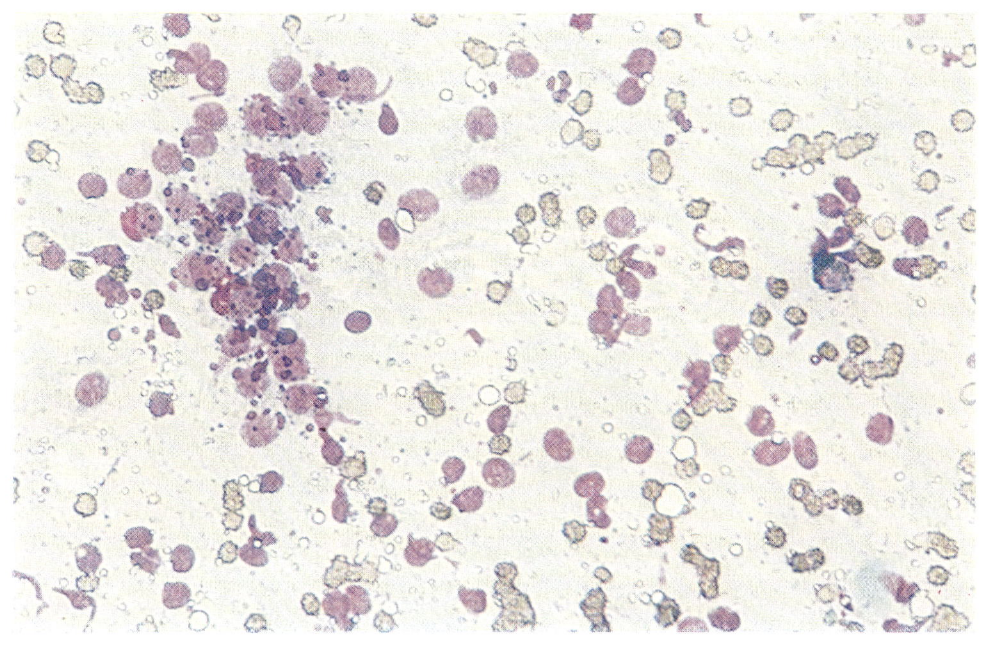

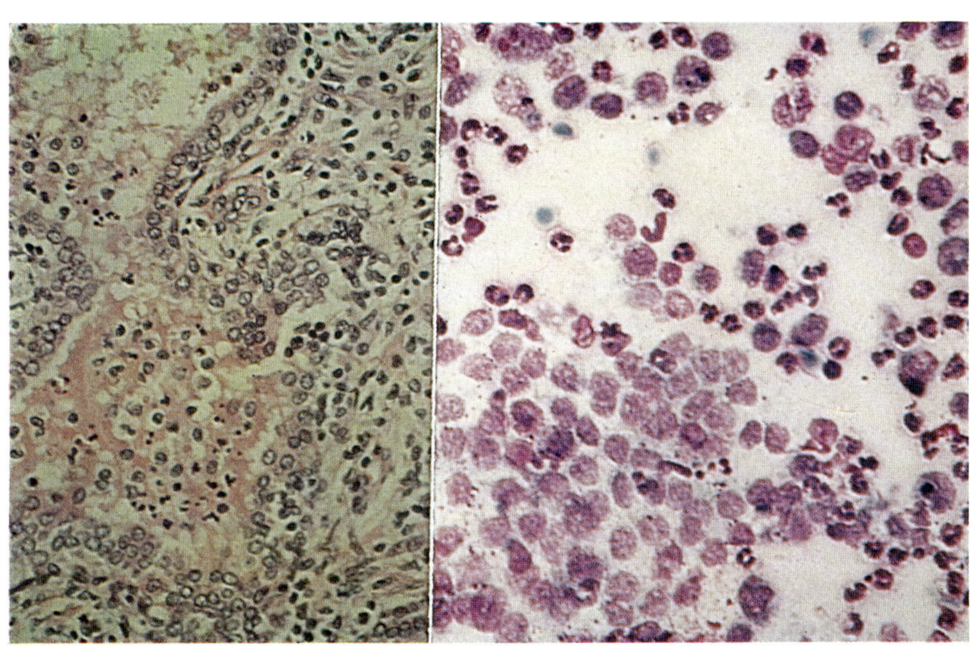

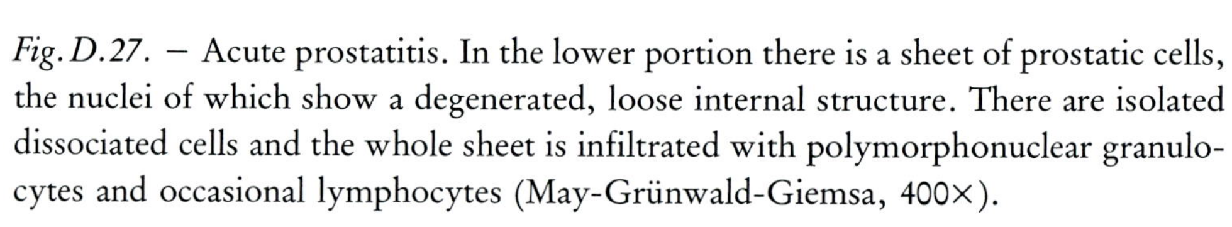

Fig. D.27. − Acute prostatitis. In the lower portion there is a sheet of prostatic cells, the nuclei of which show a degenerated, loose internal structure. There are isolated dissociated cells and the whole sheet is infiltrated with polymorphonuclear granulocytes and occasional lymphocytes (May-Grünwald-Giemsa, 400×).

Fig. D.28. − Prostatic abscess. The prostatic cells are diffusely overlaid and infiltrated by polymorphonuclear granulocytes which are multilayered in places. The slight cloudiness of the picture results from the inflammatory exudate. The slight cellular enlargement and loose appearance of the nucleoplasm are degenerative inflammatory changes (May-Grünwald-Giemsa, 400×).

56

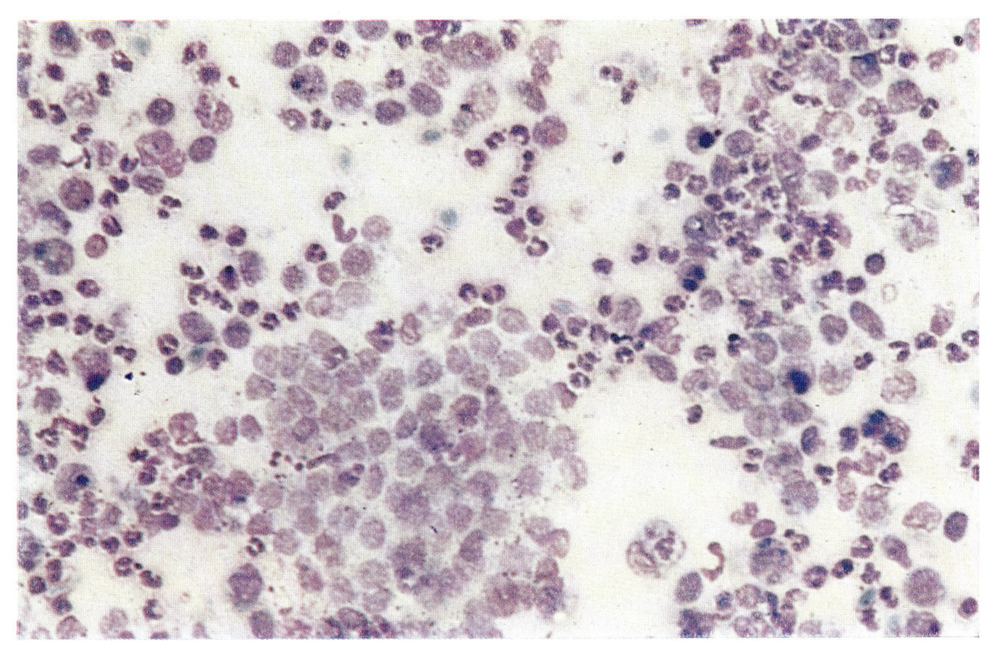

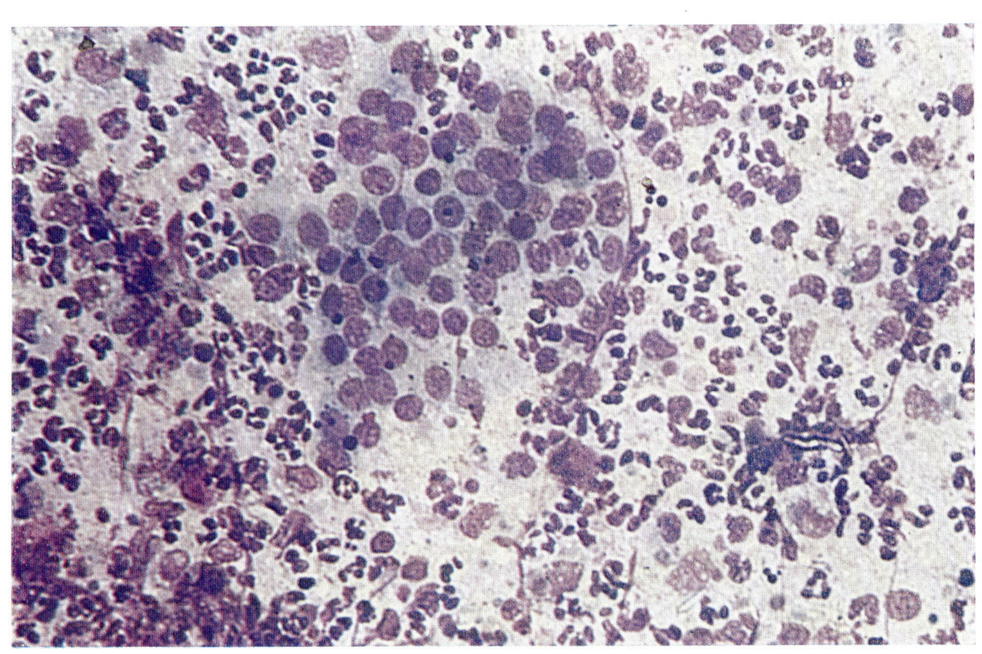

b) Chronic Prostatitis

Fig. D.29. – Chronic prostatitis. In the lower left there is a sheet of normal prostatic cells surrounded by numerous histiocytes that are recognizable by the large cytoplasmic vacuoles. Solitary lymphocytes and plasma cells are chiefly found. There are single erythrocytes and a few granulocytes (May-Grünwald-Giemsa, 400×).

Fig. D.30. – Chronic prostatitis. Sheet of normal prostatic cells surrounded by histiocytes with foamy cytoplasm. There are solitary detached prostatic cells (May-Grünwald-Giemsa, 400×).

58

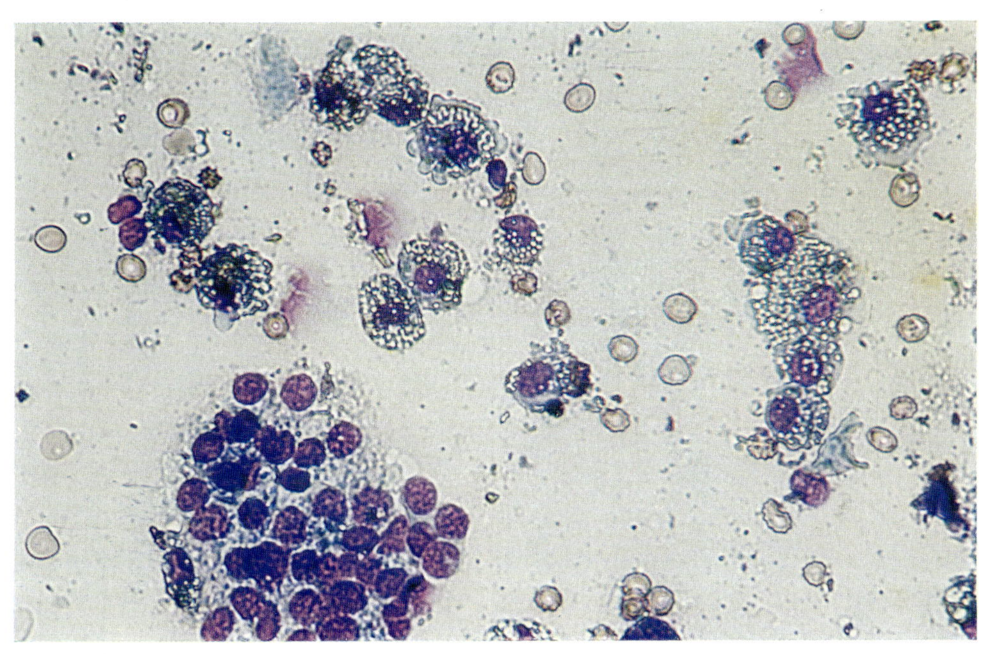

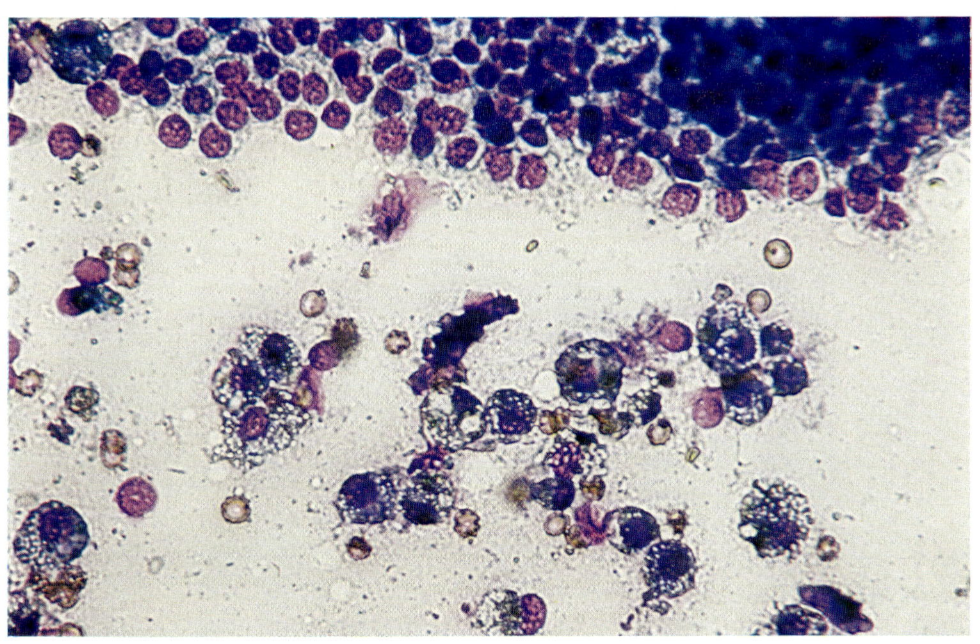

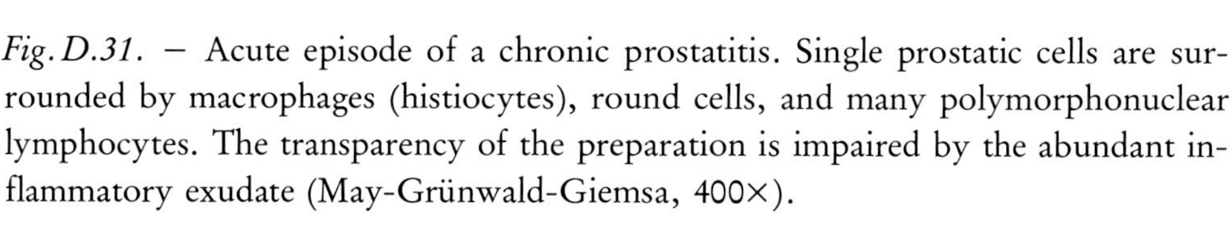

Fig. D.31. – Acute episode of a chronic prostatitis. Single prostatic cells are surrounded by macrophages (histiocytes), round cells, and many polymorphonuclear lymphocytes. The transparency of the preparation is impaired by the abundant inflammatory exudate (May-Grünwald-Giemsa, 400×).

Fig. D.32. – Subacute prostatitis. The sheet of prostatic cells shows slight inflammatory degeneration. Erythrocytes and numerous polymorphonuclear granulocytes are found in addition to round cells and histiocytes (May-Grünwald-Giemsa, 400×).

60

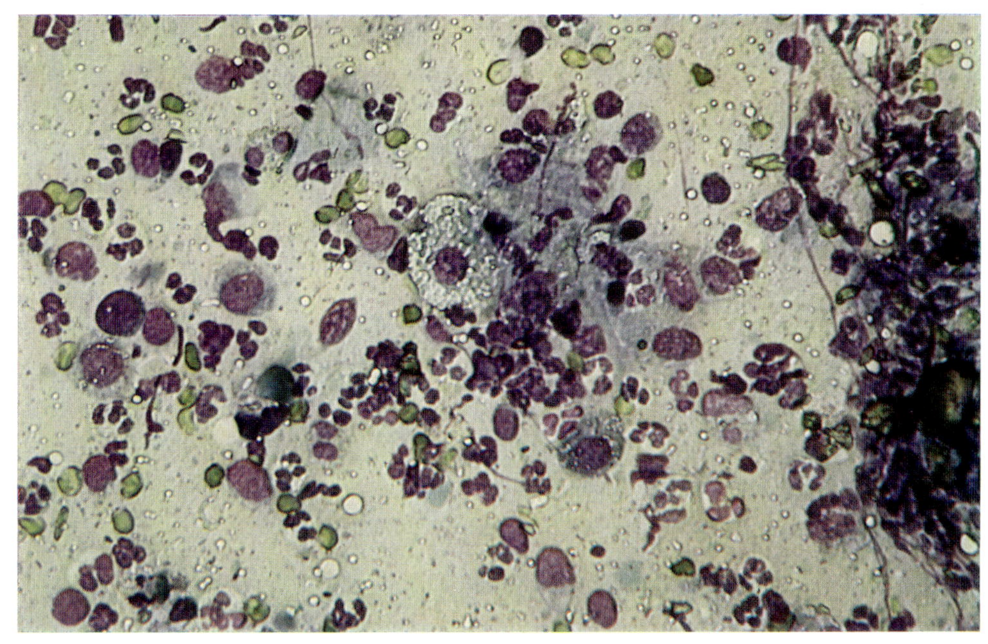

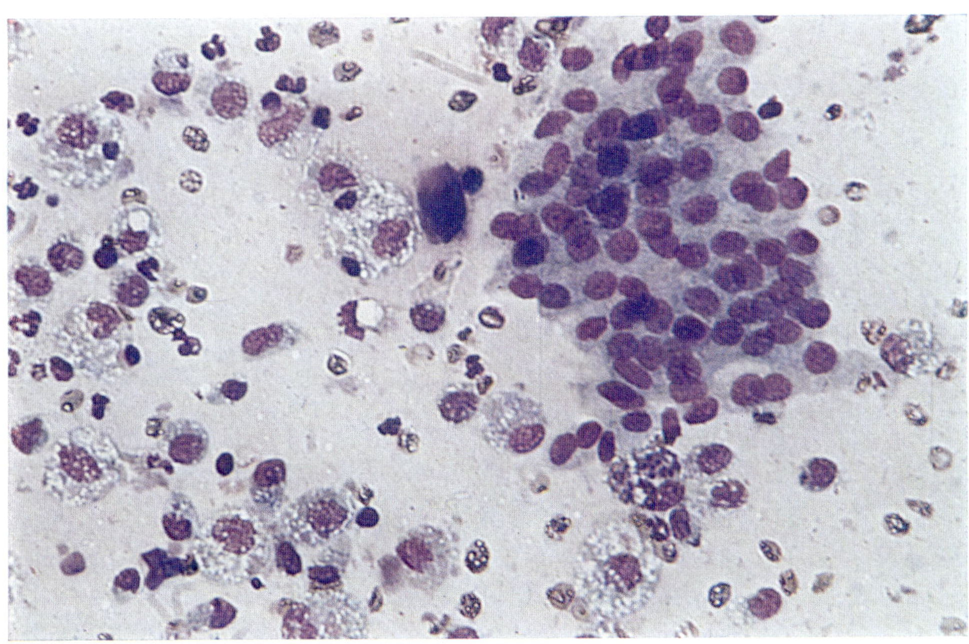

c) Granulomatous Prostatitis

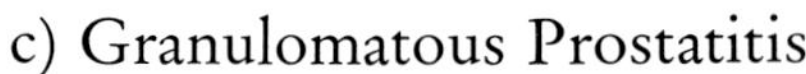

Fig.D.33. – Marked granulomatous prostatitis. In the upper right half of the picture there are prostatic cells showing inflammatory degeneration and surrounded and infiltrated with polymorphonuclear granulocytes, histiocytes, and multinucleated macrophages. Occasional eosinophilic granulocytes are also found (May-Grünwald-Giemsa, 400×).

Fig.D.34. – Granulomatous prostatitis. In addition to granulocytes, lymphocytes, and erythrocytes, there are multinucleated histiocytic giant cells with centrally placed nuclei. To the right are seen degenrate, inflamed prostatic cells (May-Grünwald-Giemsa, 400×).

62

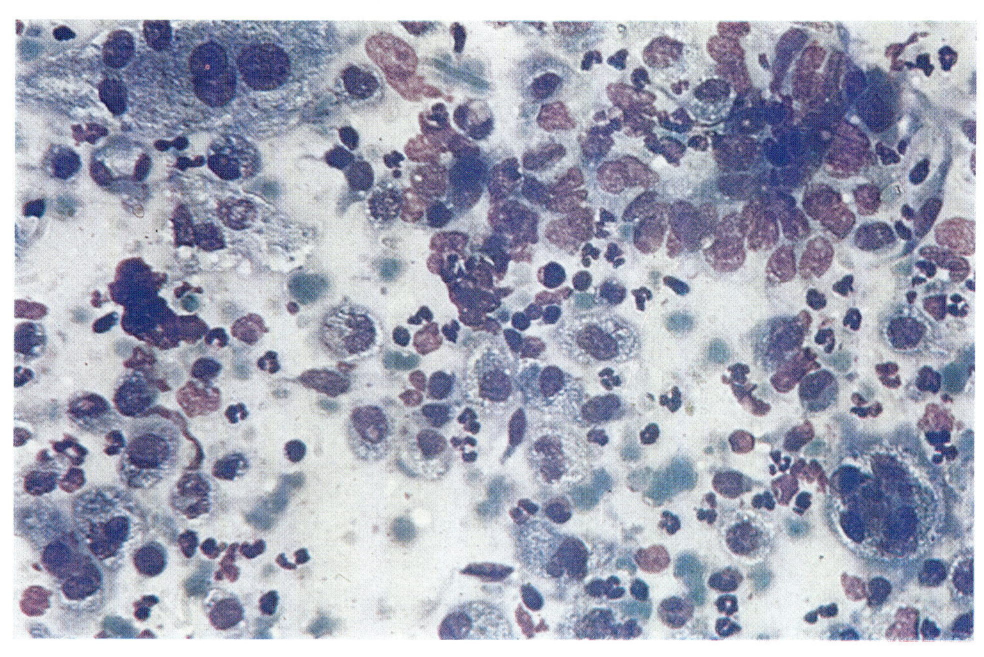

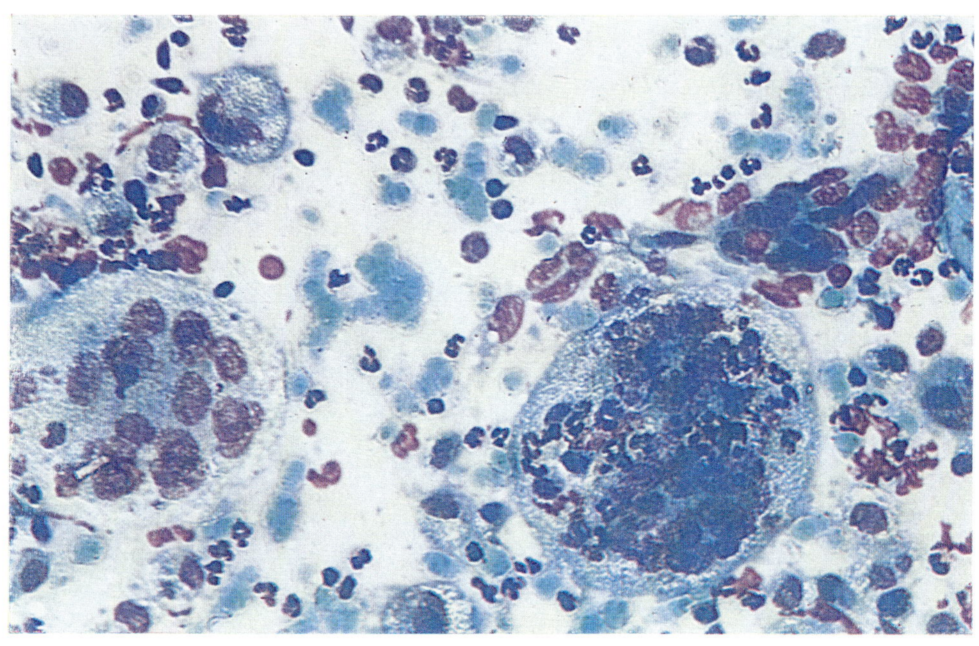

Fig. D.35. – Solitary multinucleated giant cell ("granuloma cell"). The cytoplasm is not only vacuolated, but it is also strongly basophilic. The sheet of prostatic cells appears to be somewhat loosely attached. The nucleoplasm shows slight edematous swelling (May-Grünwald-Giemsa, 400×).

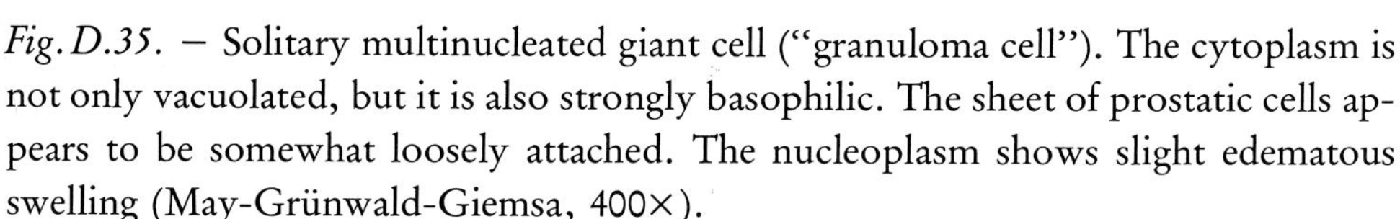

Fig. D.36. – Granulomatous prostatitis with marked degenerative changes of the prostatic epithelial cells, which are surrounded by many granuloma cells, leukocytes, lymphocytes, and erythrocytes. In the center the sheet of prostatic cells is multilayered and overlaid with cells and therefore indistinct. The smear appears decidedly cloudy probably because of the inflammatory exudate (May-Grünwald-Giemsa, 400×).

64

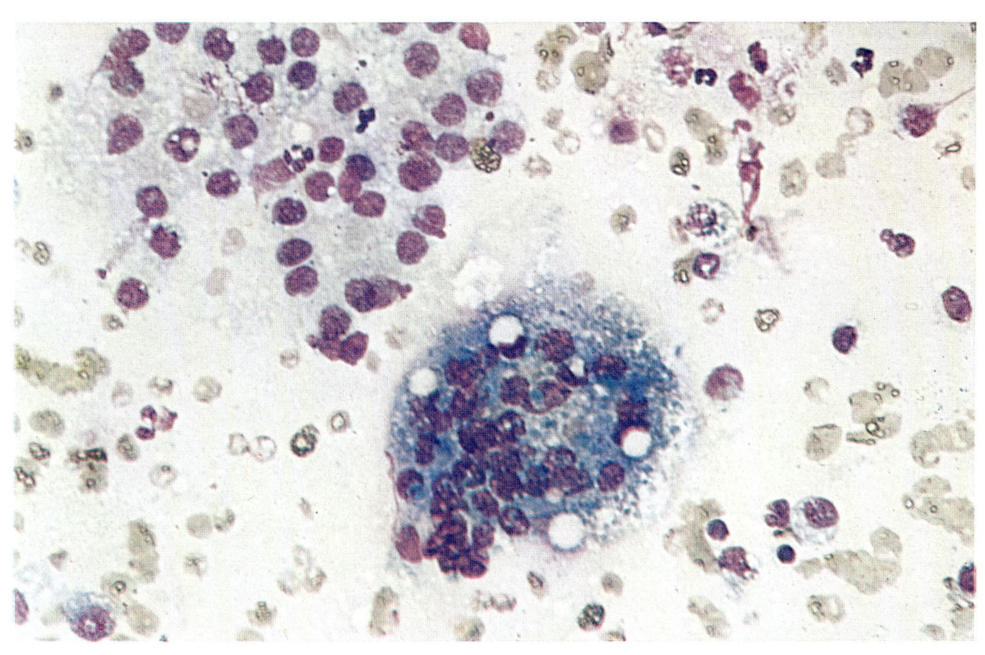

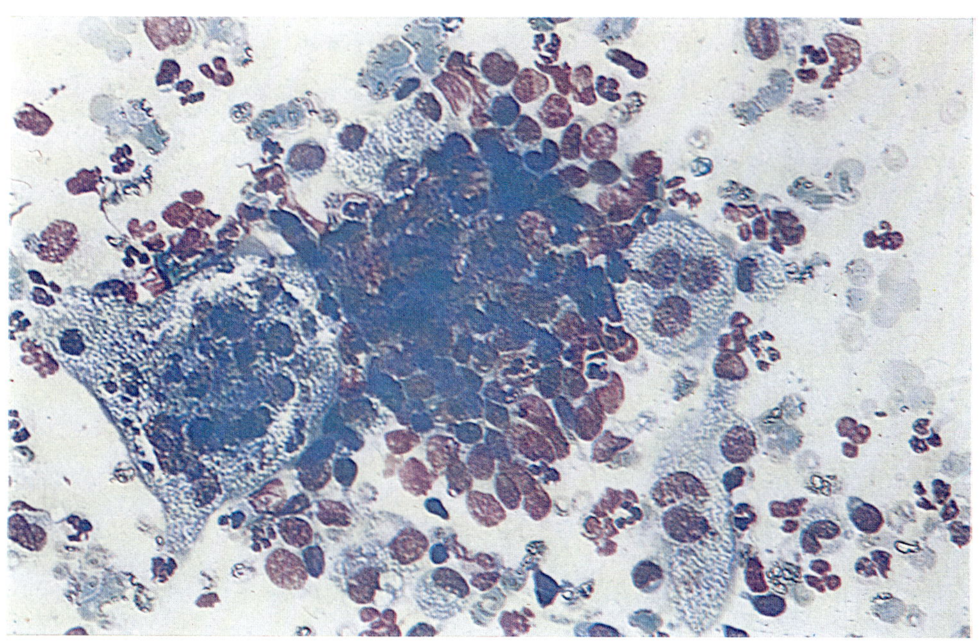

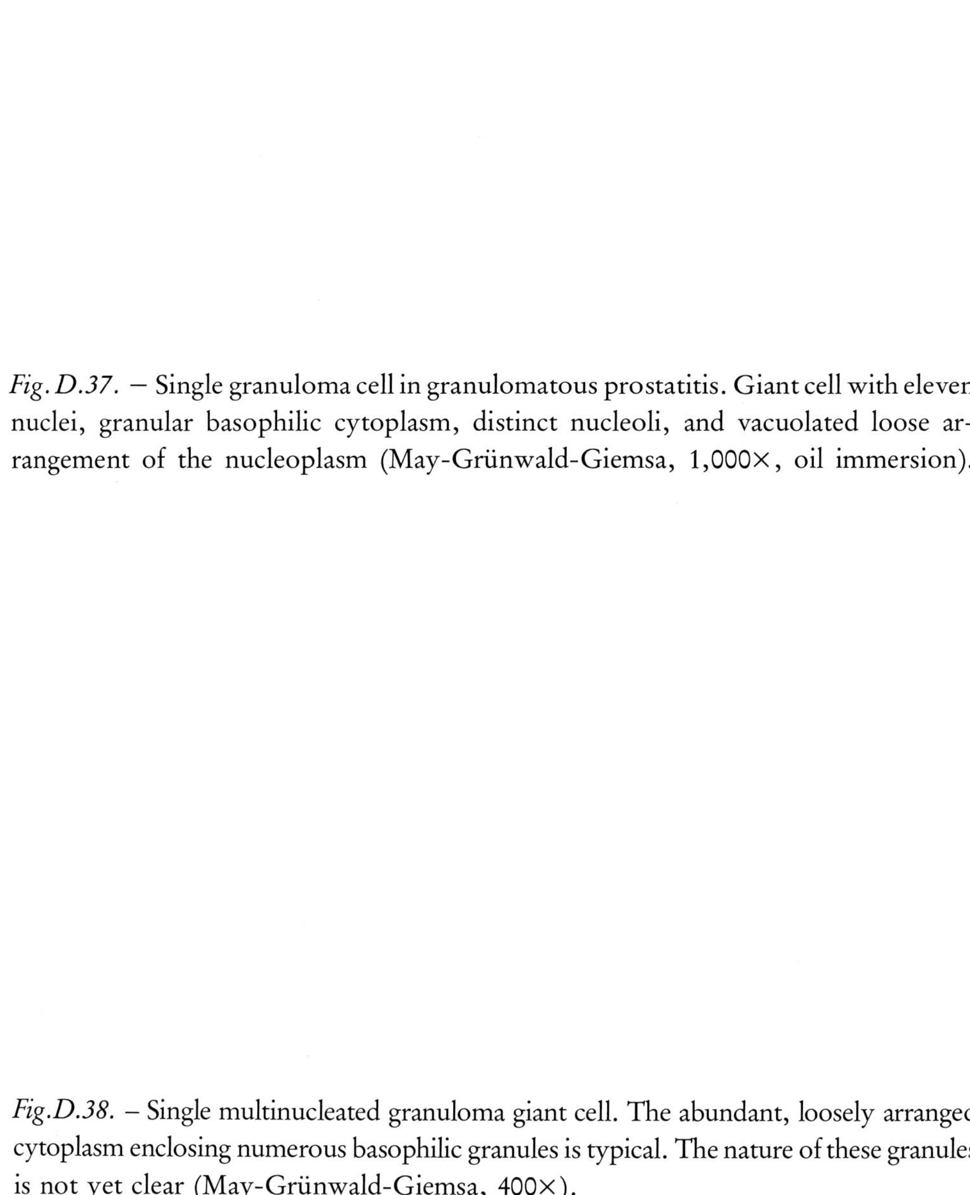

Fig. D.37. – Single granuloma cell in granulomatous prostatitis. Giant cell with eleven nuclei, granular basophilic cytoplasm, distinct nucleoli, and vacuolated loose arrangement of the nucleoplasm (May-Grünwald-Giemsa, 1,000×, oil immersion).

Fig.D.38. – Single multinucleated granuloma giant cell. The abundant, loosely arranged cytoplasm enclosing numerous basophilic granules is typical. The nature of these granules is not yet clear (May-Grünwald-Giemsa, 400×).

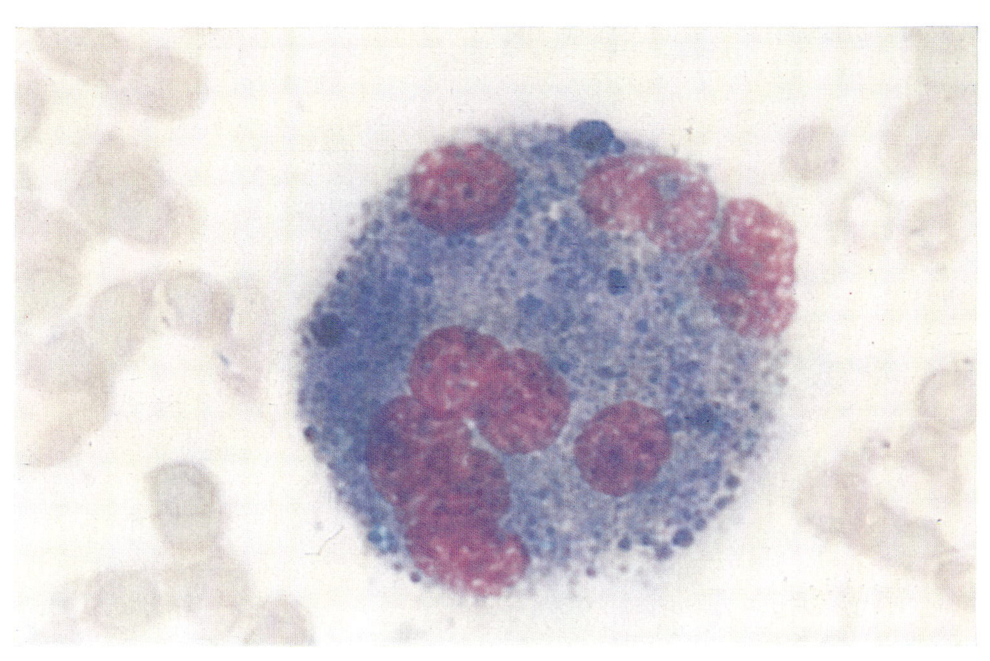

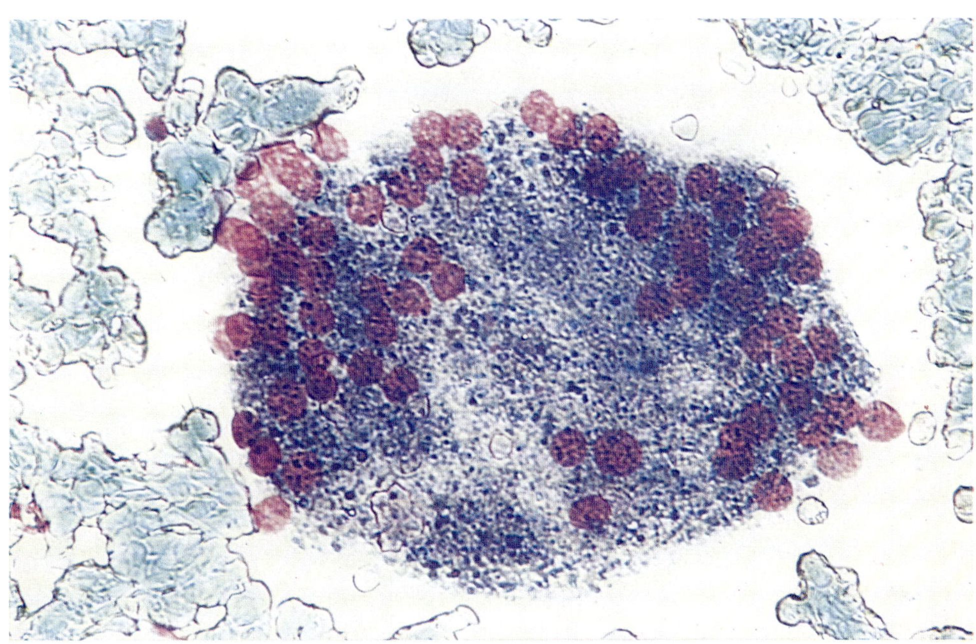

Fig.D.39. – Severe granulomatous prostatitis in a moderately well-differentiated prostatic carcinoma. One should always be suspicious that a carcinoma may arise in granulomatous prostatitis. A careful search must be made in such cases for evidences of malignancy, and if the smear is negative another biopsy should be taken after three months (May-Grünwald-Giemsa, 400×).

3. Carcinoma of the Prostate

a) Well-Differentiated Carcinoma

Fig.D.40. – Simultaneous biopsies of a well-differentiated adenocarcinoma of the prostate. On the *left* is the histologic preparation. In some parts there are groups of highly differentiated cells and in other parts there are small numbers of undifferentiated cells typically showing nuclear pleomorphism and large nucleoli (HE, 250×). On the *right* is the cytologic preparation from the same patient. The nuclear polymorphism and polychromasia are far beyond normal limits. The pattern of the cell sheet is much altered and there are hyperchromatic, pyknotic malignant cells, some of which have prominent nucleoli (HE, 250×).

68

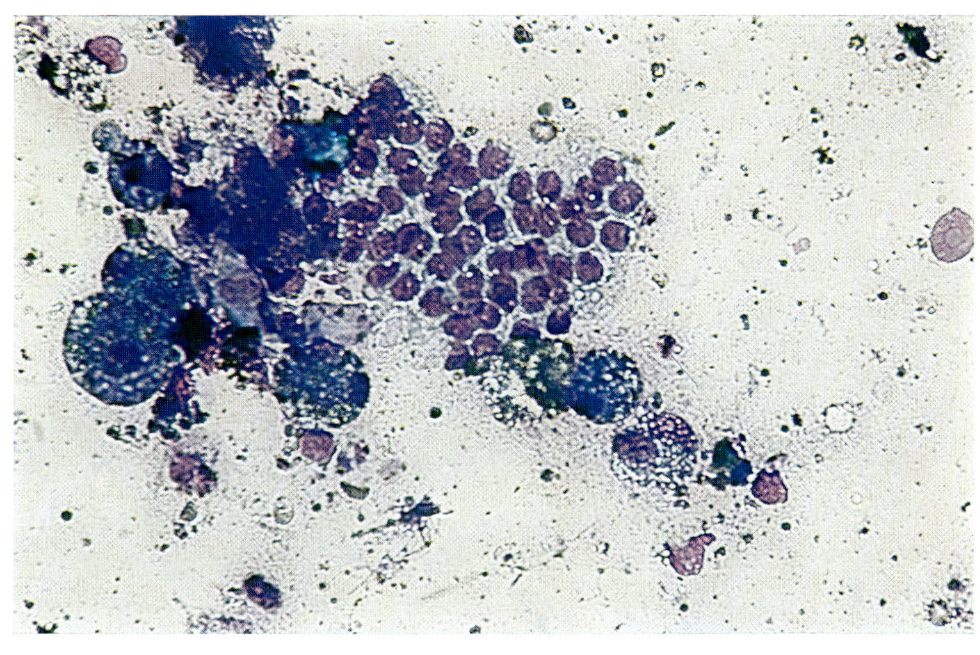

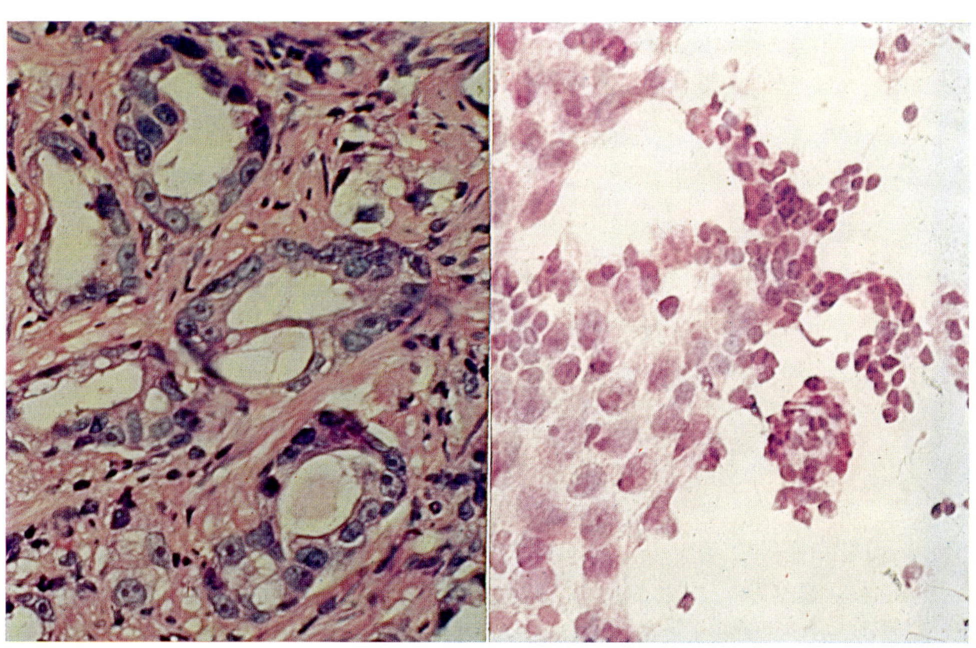

Fig.D.41. – Cytologically well-differentiated adenocarcinoma of the prostate. The festoonlike arrangement of the cell nuclei, frequently without cell borders, is pathognomonic. Such acini are found throughout the entire smear (May-Grünwald-Giemsa, 400×).

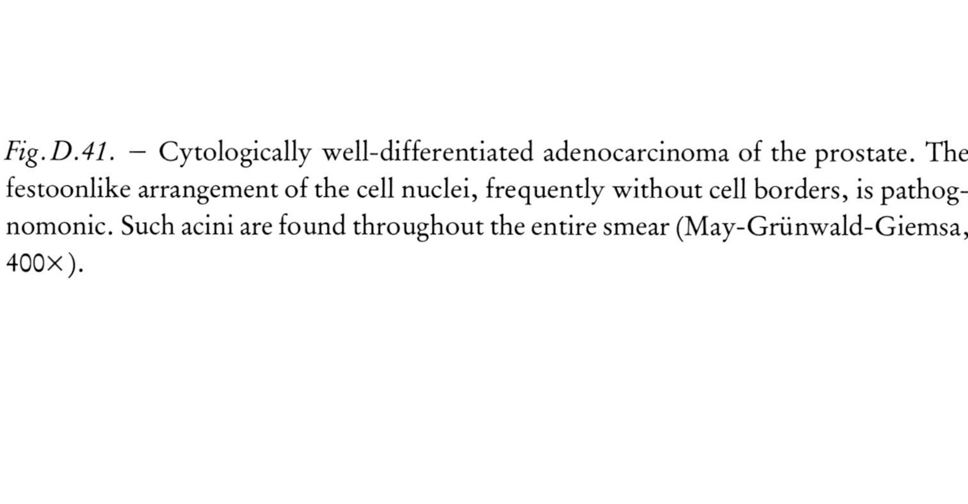

Fig.D.42. – So-called microadenoma – a pseudoacinar arrangement of tumor cell nuclei around centrally situated cytoplasm showing no cell borders (May-Grünwald-Giemsa, 100×, oil immersion).

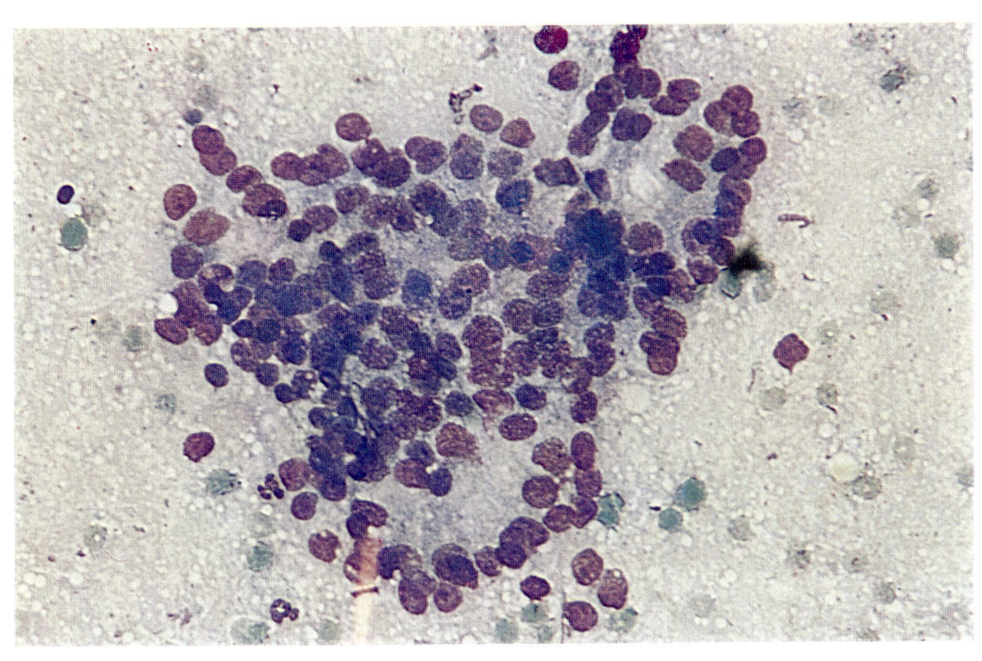

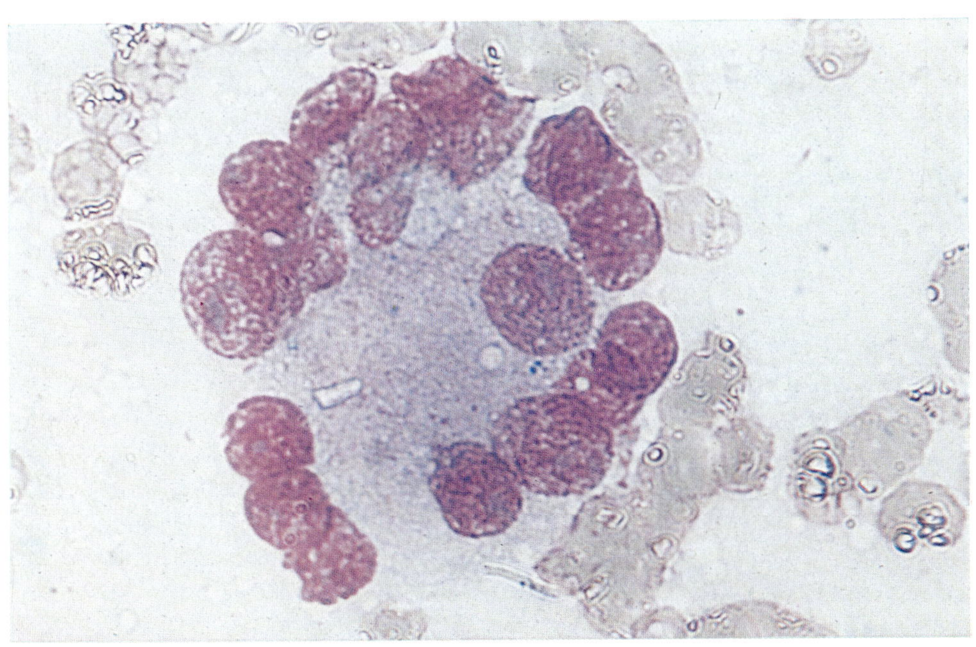

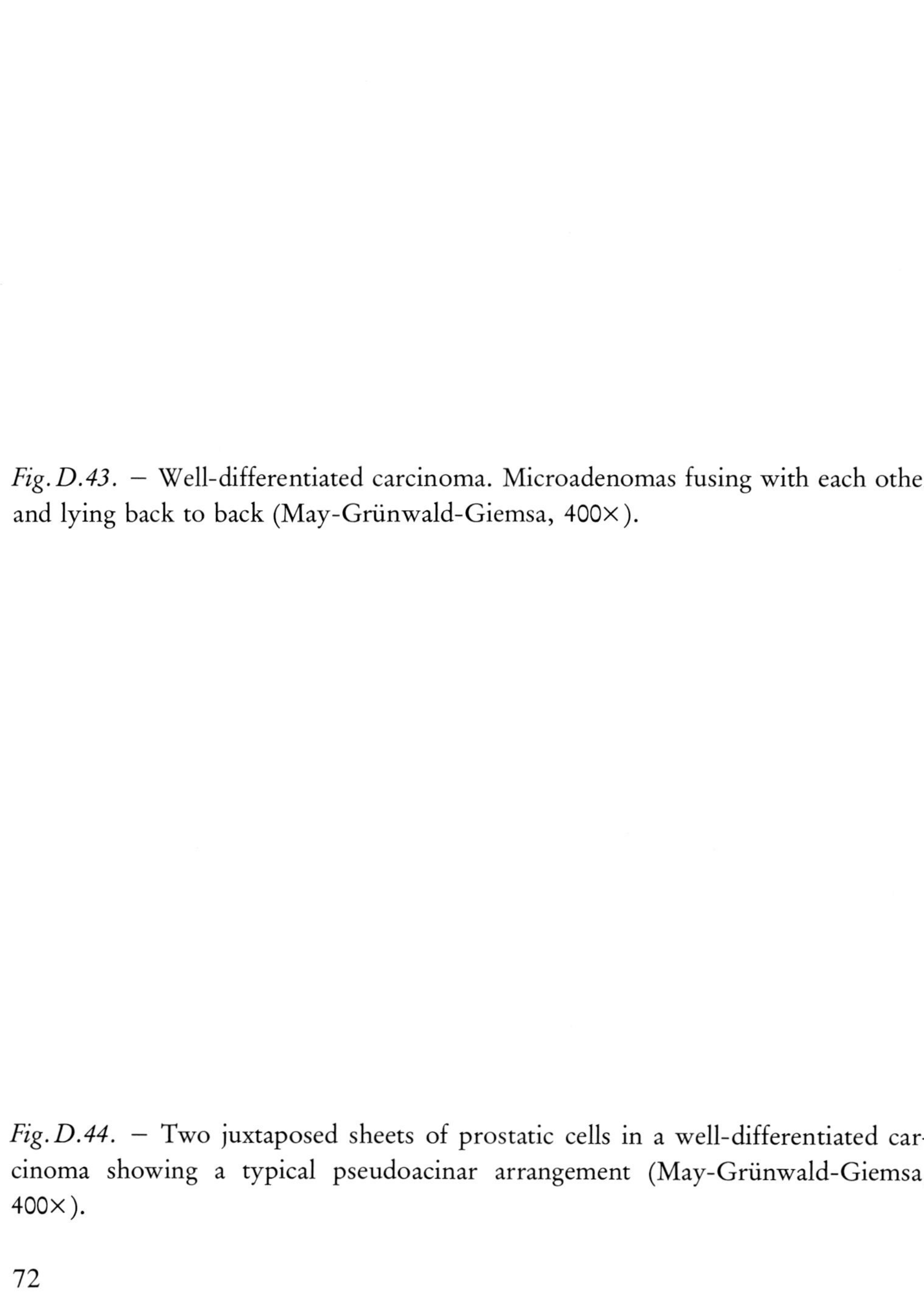

Fig.D.43. – Well-differentiated carcinoma. Microadenomas fusing with each other and lying back to back (May-Grünwald-Giemsa, 400×).

Fig.D.44. – Two juxtaposed sheets of prostatic cells in a well-differentiated carcinoma showing a typical pseudoacinar arrangement (May-Grünwald-Giemsa, 400×).

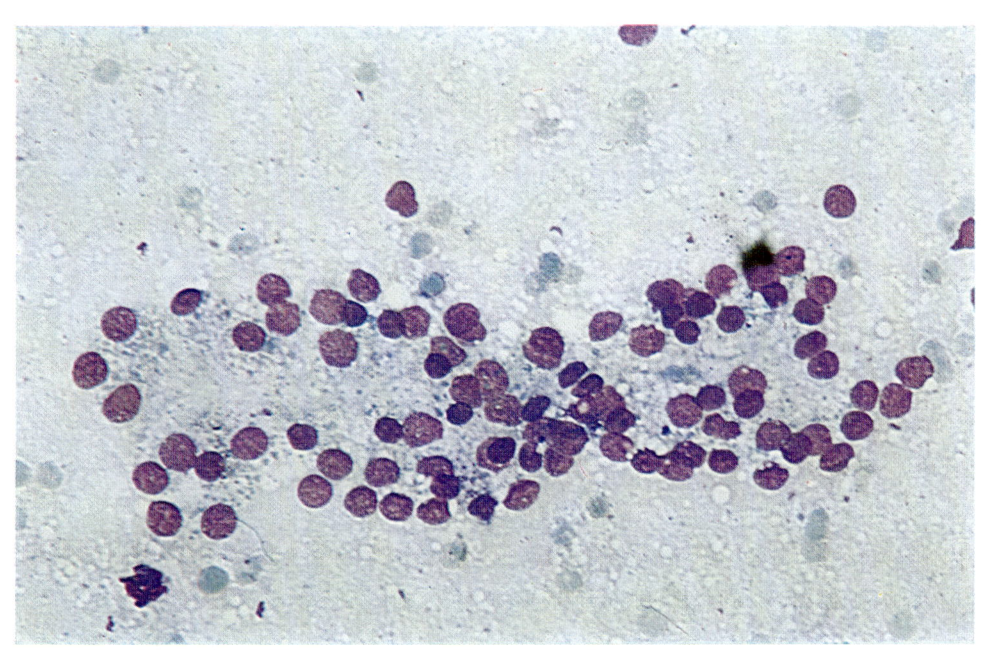

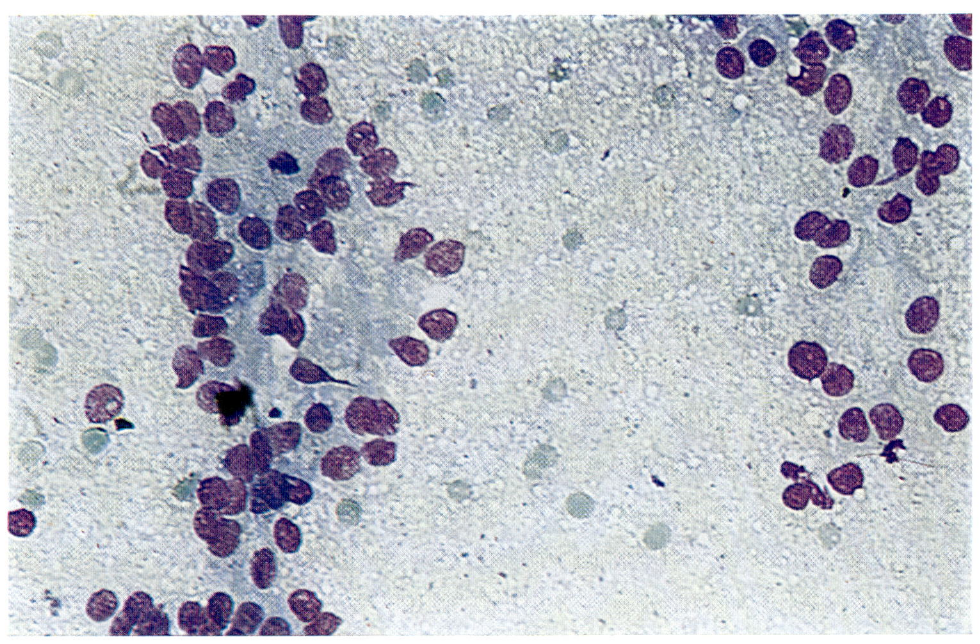

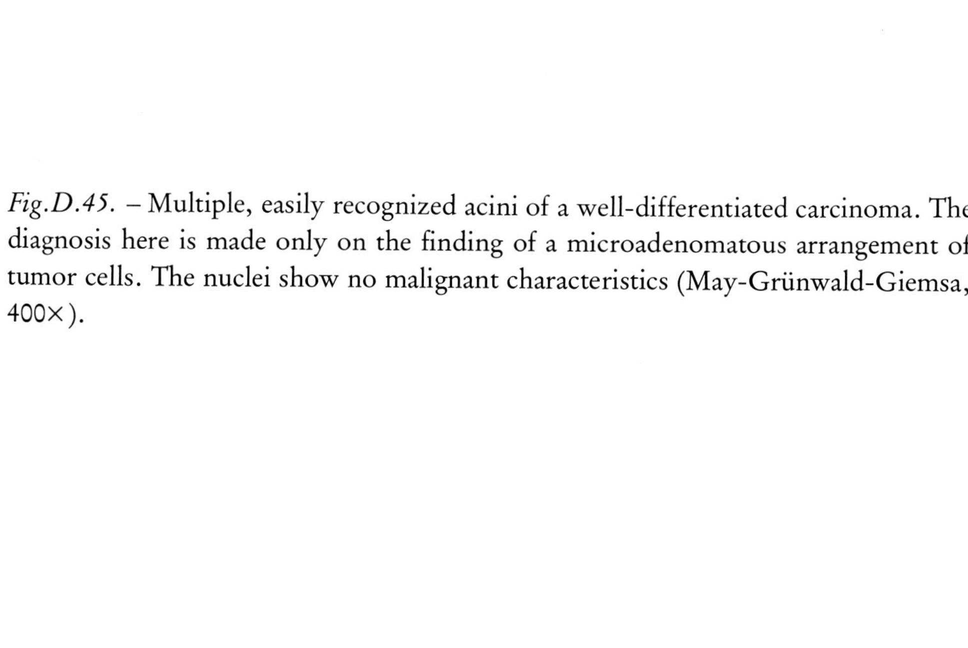

Fig.D.45. – Multiple, easily recognized acini of a well-differentiated carcinoma. The diagnosis here is made only on the finding of a microadenomatous arrangement of tumor cells. The nuclei show no malignant characteristics (May-Grünwald-Giemsa, 400×).

Fig.D.46. – Well-differentiated carcinoma. Sheet of cells with connecting acini. Slight anisonucleosis and absence of cell borders (May-Grünwald-Giemsa, 400×).

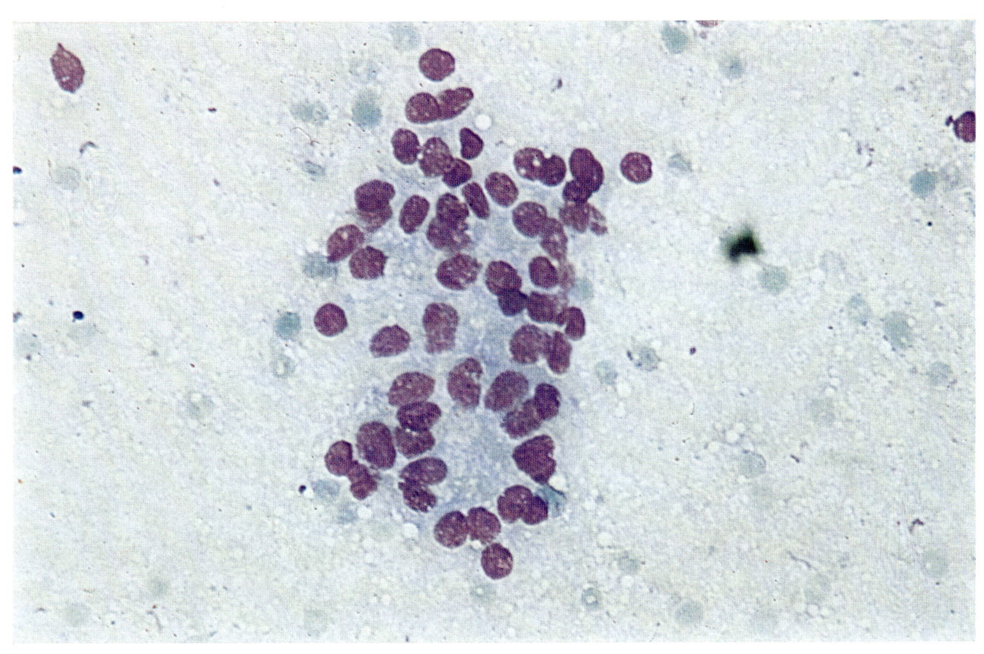

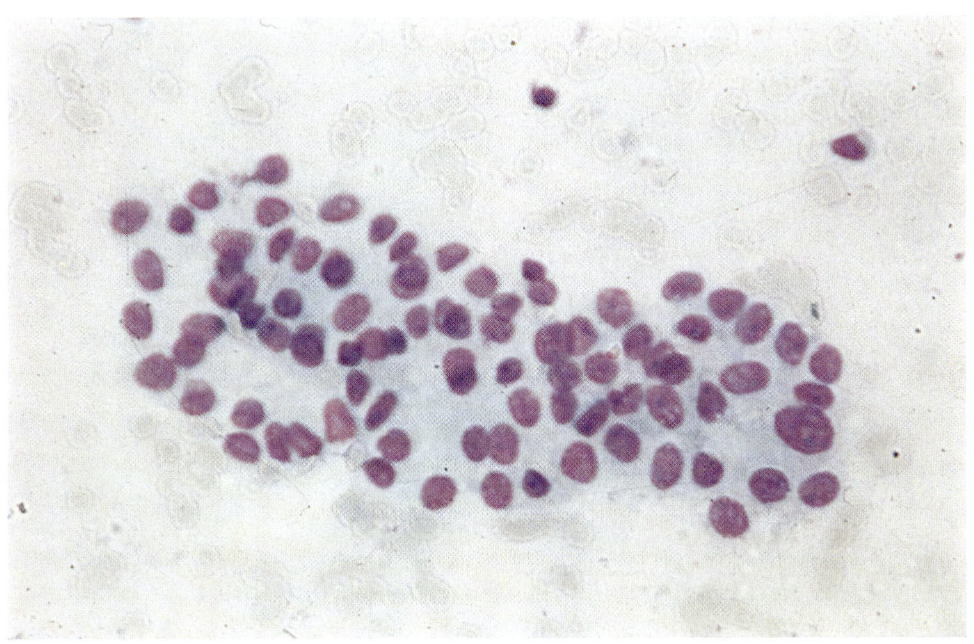

b) Moderately Well-Differentiated Carcinoma

Fig. D.47. – Simultaneous biopsies of a moderately well-differentiated carcinoma of the prostate. On the *left* is the histologic preparation. This less well-differentiated tumor is growing in solid nests with only here and there a recognizable adenomatous structure (HE, 250×). On the *right* is the cytologic preparation. There are loosely adherent aggregates and free lying solitary nuclei. The prominent, large nucleoli and clumped chromatin pattern are typical (May-Grünwald-Giemsa, 400×).

Fig. D.48. – Sheet of normal prostatic cells in the lower right corner; above it are large tumor cells with prominent nucleoli from a moderately well-differentiated carcinoma. The cells have a microacinar arrangement and are without recognizable cytoplasmic margins (May-Grünwald-Giemsa, 400×).

76

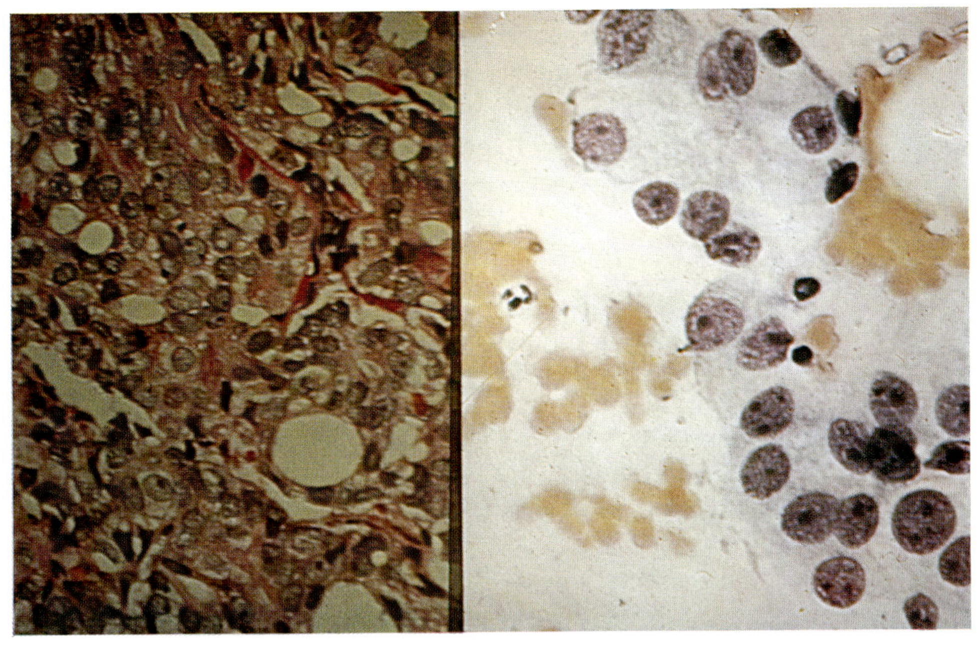

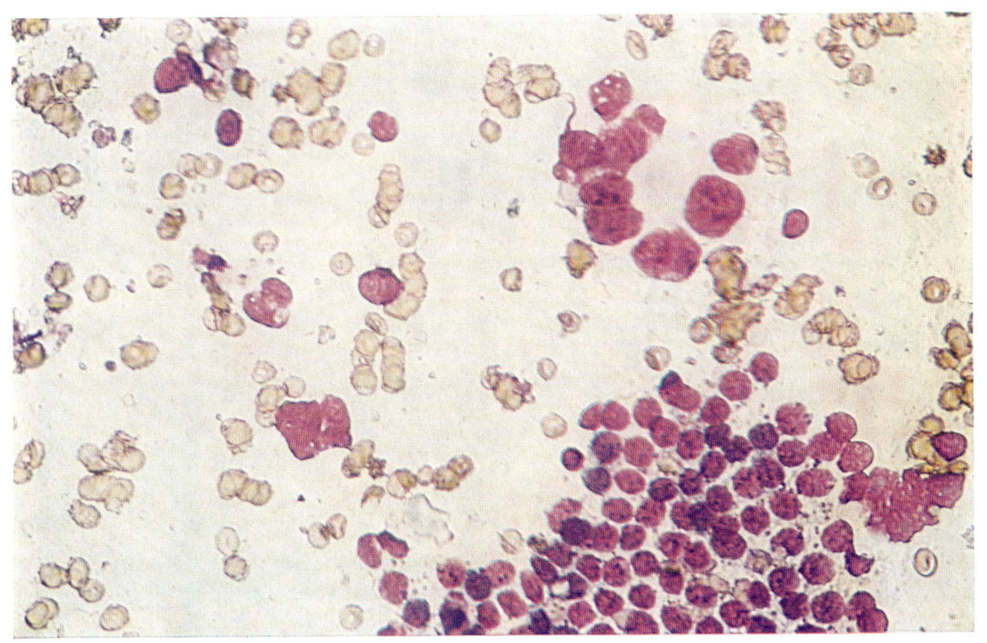

Fig.D.49. − Loosely bound aggregates of tumor cells from a moderately well-differentiated carcinoma of the prostate. The prominent nucleoli, as many as four per
nucleus, are striking. The dissociated appearance of the aggregate can be plainly seen as
well as the free-lying, single nuclei of some tumor cells (May-Grünwald-Giemsa,
400×).

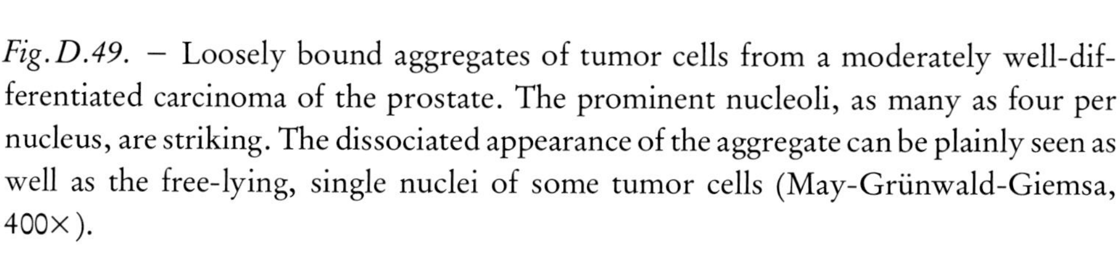

Fig.D.50. − Moderately well-differentiated prostatic carcinoma showing overlapping
of cells. There is marked nuclear polymorphism with impressive nucleoli in large nuclei (May-Grünwald-Giemsa, 400×).

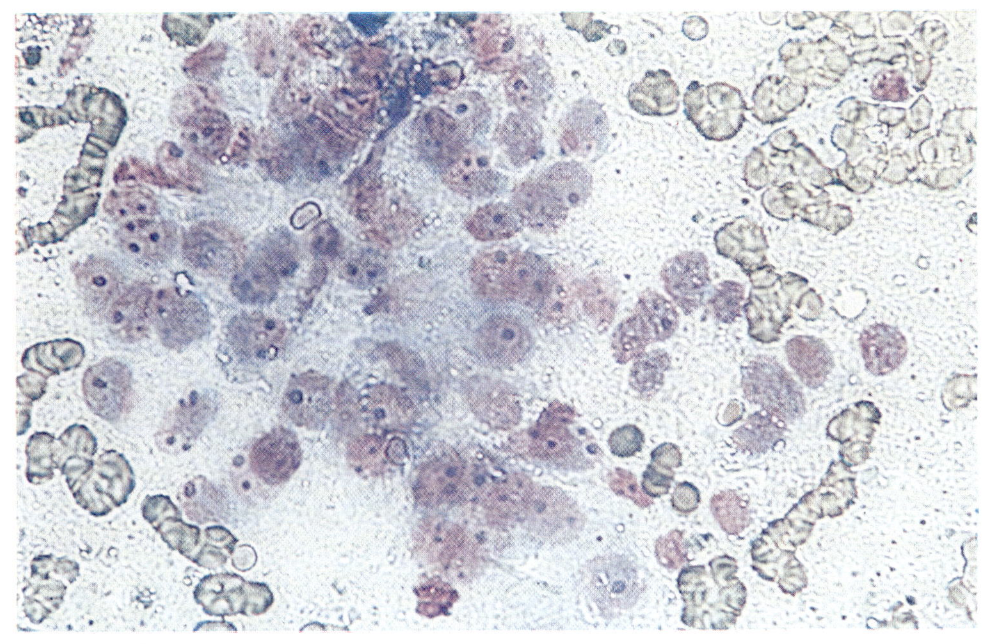

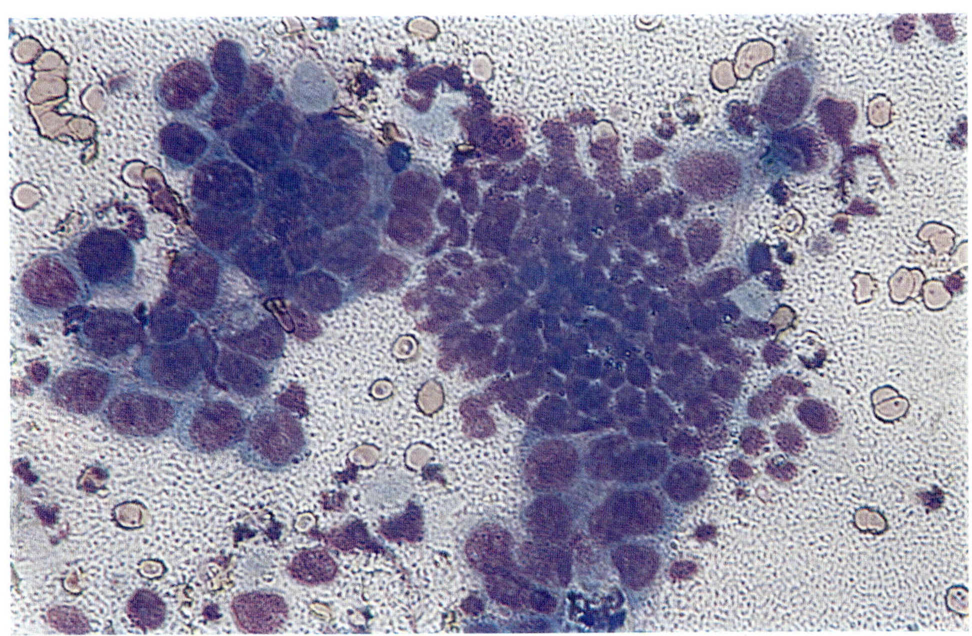

Fig.D.51. – Moderately well-differentiated prostatic carcinoma with marked dissociation of tumor cells and anisonucleosis. Hyperchromasia and polymorphism are striking (Papanicolaou, 400×).

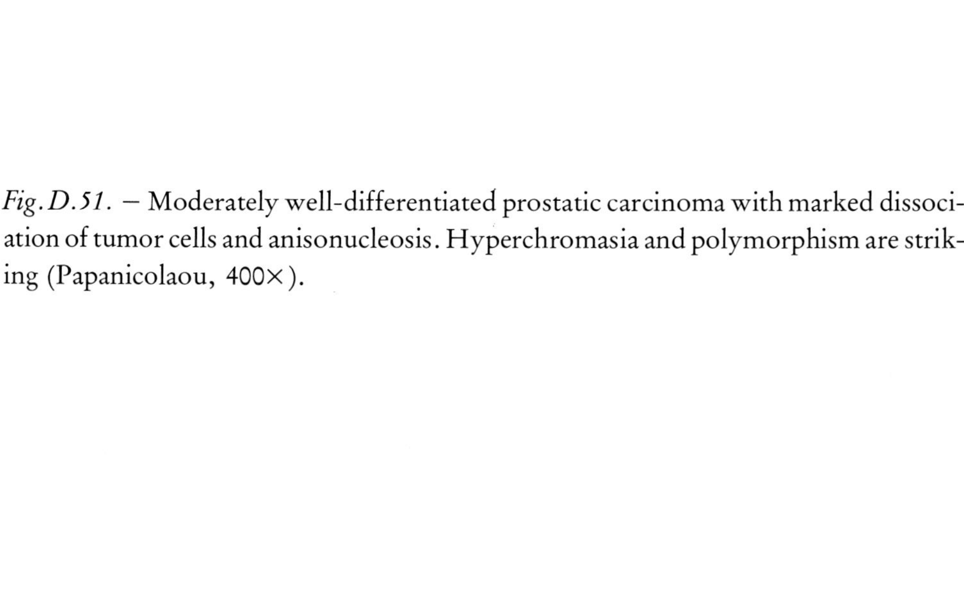

Fig.D.52. – Moderately well-differentiaded carcinoma of the prostate. Partial dissociation of the sheet arrangement with only loose binding of the cells. Cytoplasmic borders can no longer be recognized, nuclear polymorphism and polychromasia are marked, and there are clearly visible nucleoli in almost all nuclei (May-Grünwald-Giemsa, 1,000×, oil immersion).

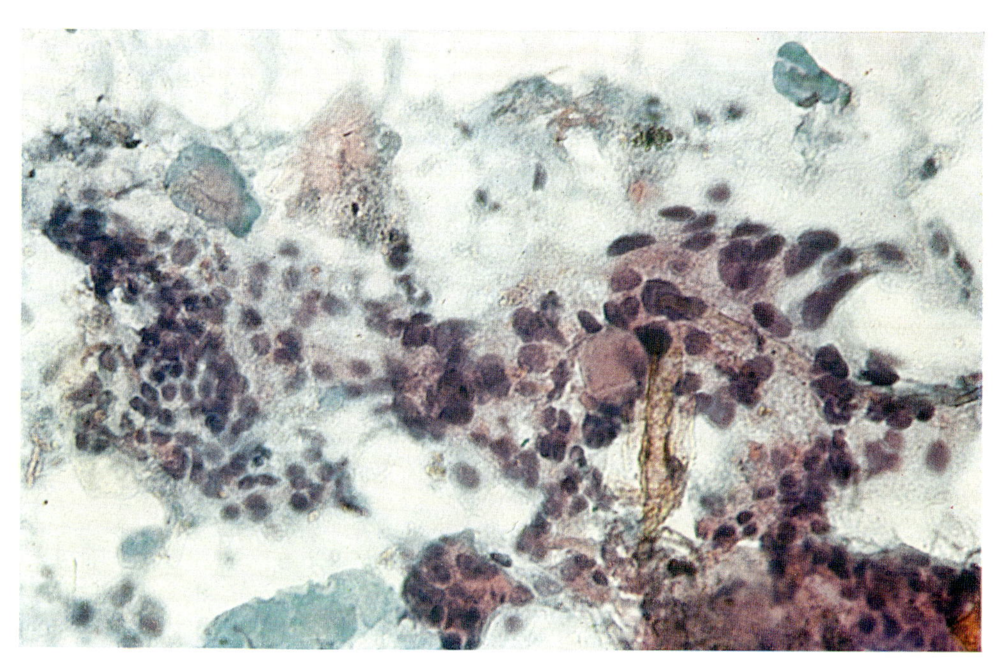

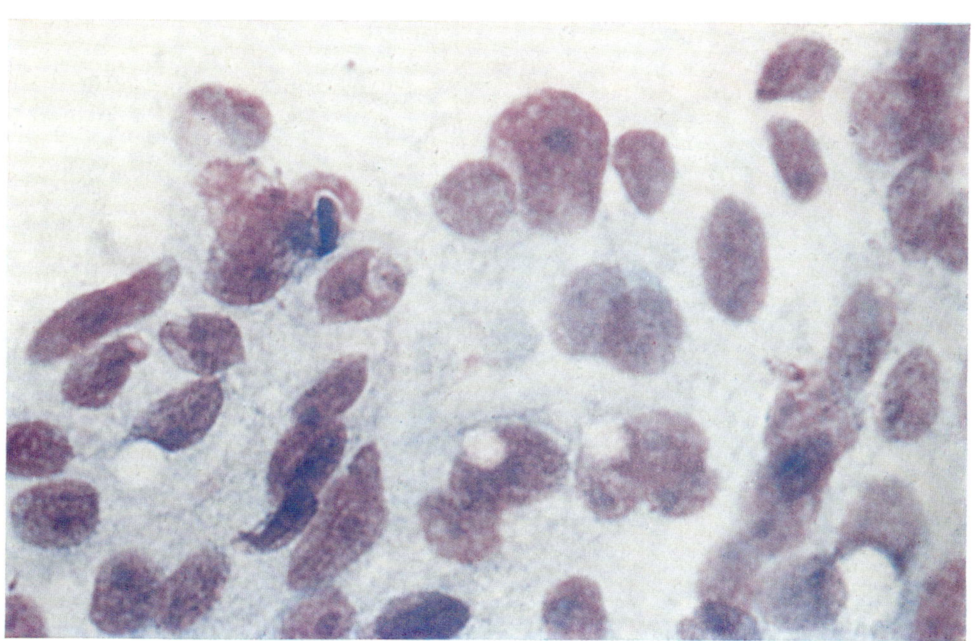

Fig. D.53. – At the lower margin of the picture there are normal prostatic cells showing partial overlapping. Above them lies a sheet of atypical nuclei that at the upper
margin of the picture shows distinct large nucleoli and the features of a moderately
well-differentiated prostatic carcinoma (May-Grünwald-Giemsa, 400×).

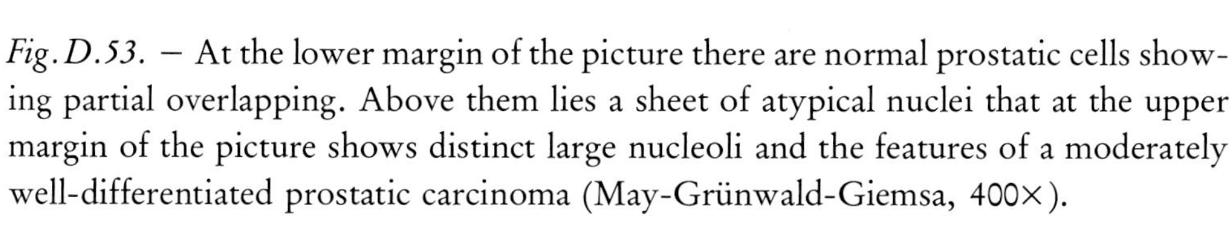

Fig. D.54. – Moderately well-differentiated prostatic carcinoma. Many of the nuclei
overlap one another in multiple layers, making differentiation difficult. The multiple
nucleoli can be clearly seen. There is no longer an orderly sheetlike arrangement of the
cells (May-Grünwald-Giemsa, 1,000×, oil immersion).

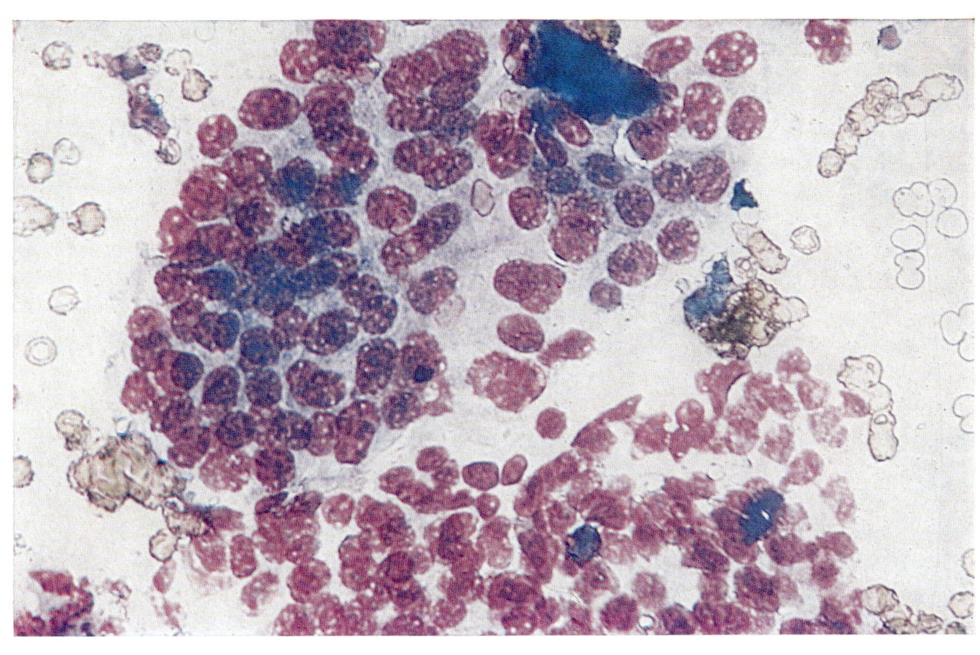

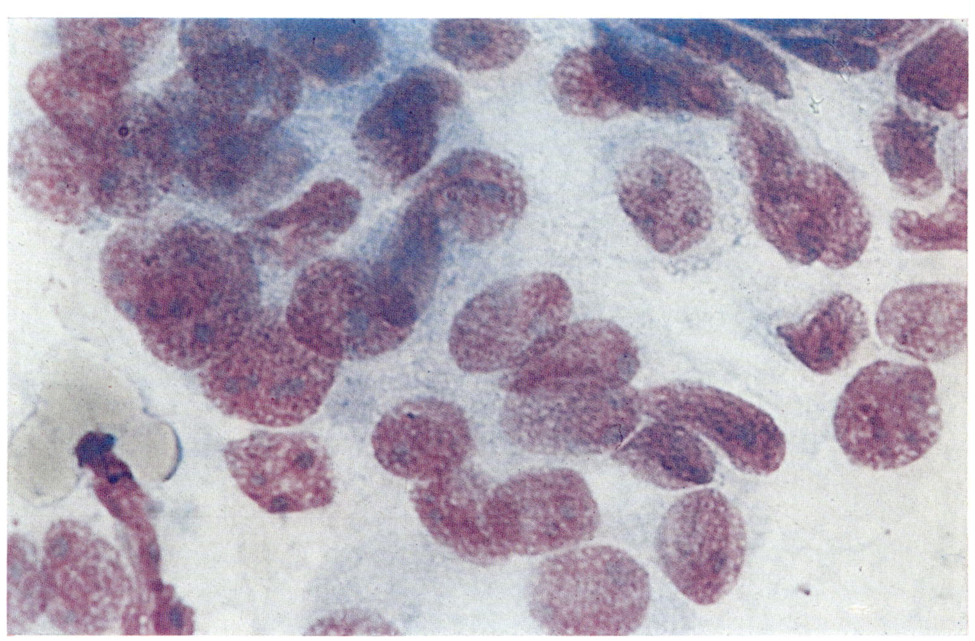

Fig. D.55. – Moderately differentiated prostatic carcinoma. A sheetlike pattern is still partially preserved. The apparent abundance of nuclei is chiefly due to overlapping of cells that show more than normal polymorphism and polychromasia. Some tumor cells are partly dissociated and have single large nucleoli (May-Grünwald-Giemsa, 400×).

c) Undifferentiated Carcinoma

Fig. D.56. – Simultaneous biopsies of an undifferentiated prostatic carcinoma. *Left,* the histologic preparation: the tumor forms small, solid nests and strands of cells having no recognizable glandular pattern. Polymorphism is marked (HE, 250×). *Right,* the cytologic preparation: there are free-lying single nuclei without any sheet arrangement, marked polymorphism and polychromasia, and many large prominent nucleoli. This is from a patient already under estrogen treatment, so there is marked vacuolation of the nucleoplasm (May-Grünwald-Giemsa, 1,000×, oil immersion).

84

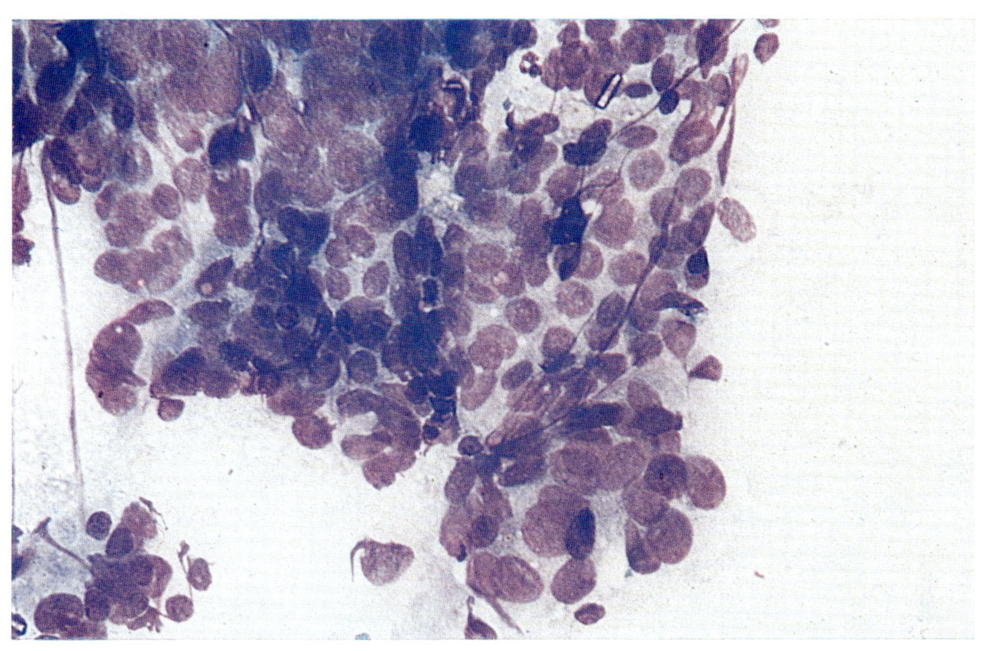

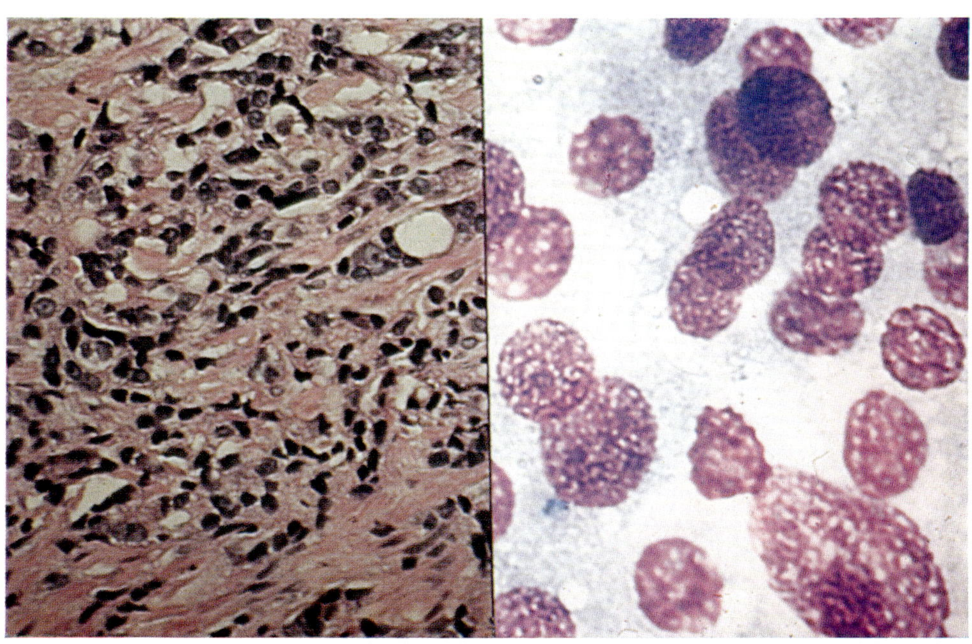

Fig.D.57. – Undifferentiated prostatic carcinoma. Dissociated, free-lying nuclei showing very marked polymorphism and scarcely recognizable cytoplasm. The fragmentation and squeezing of nuclei are artifacts due to increased fragility of the tumor cells (on the left side of the picture, May-Grünwald-Giemsa, 1,000×, oil immersion).

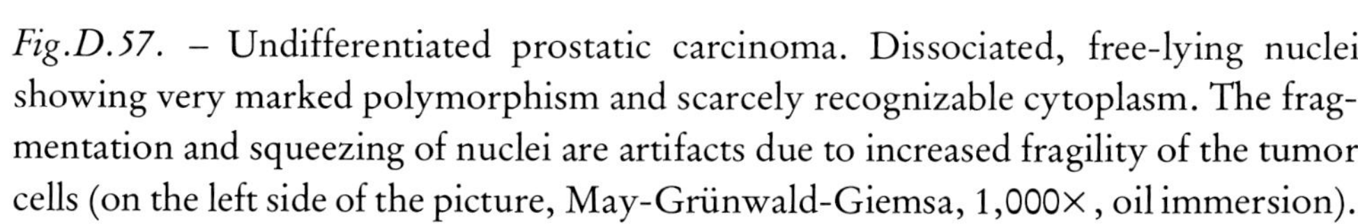

Fig.D.58. – Undifferentiated carcinoma of the prostate. The free-lying, isolated nuclei and the formation of aggregates of large, bizarre nuclei are typical. Cytoplasmic borders are no longer preserved (May-Grünwald-Giemsa, 1,000×, oil immersion).

86

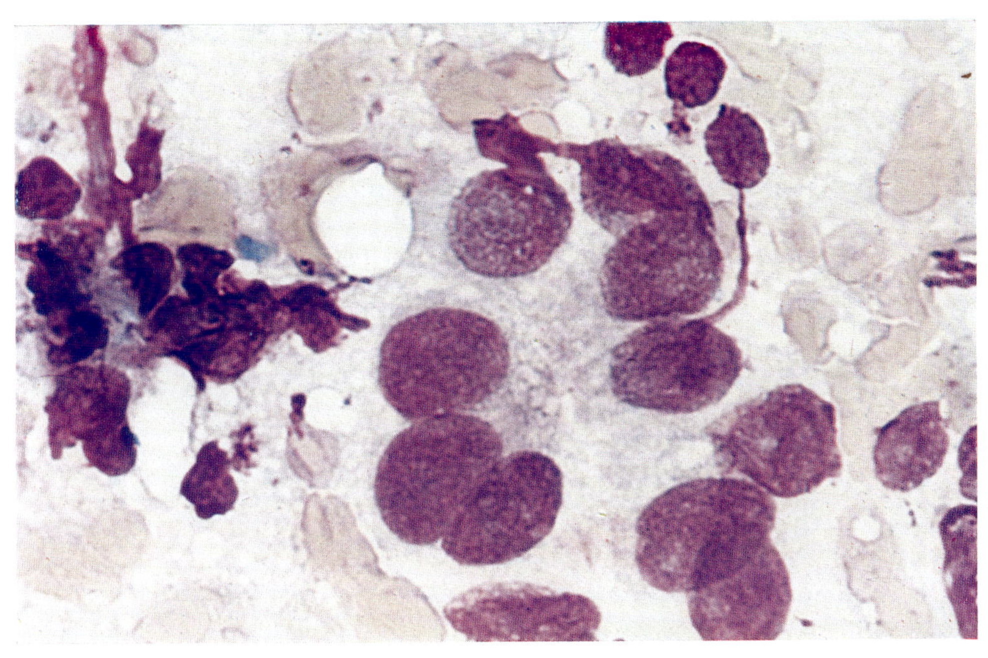

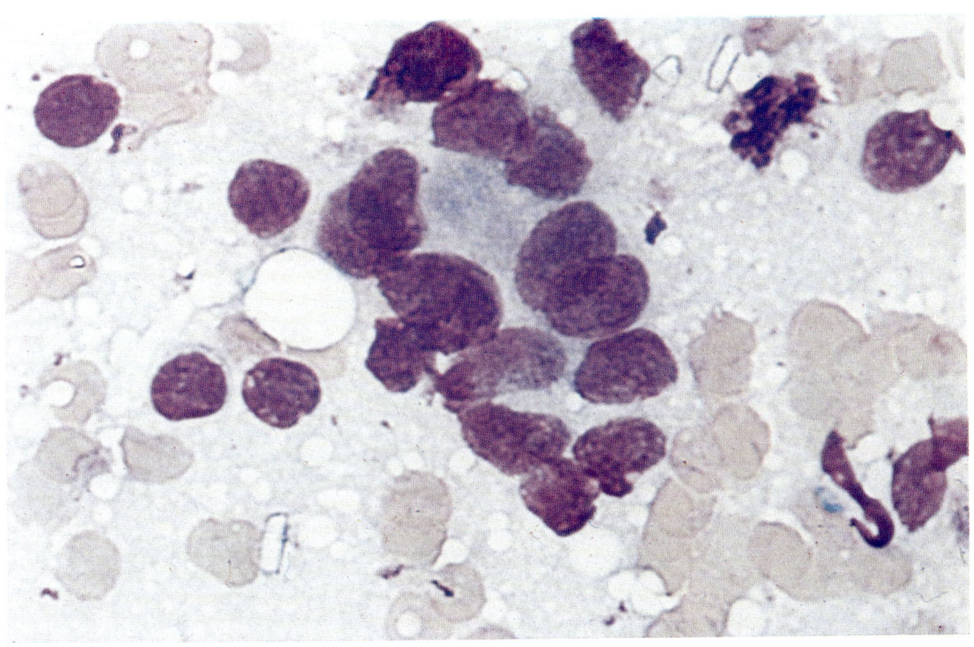

Fig.D.59. – Undifferentiated prostatic carcinoma. There is still a suggestion of an aggregate pattern, but polymorphism is extreme and the ratio of nucleus to plasma is shifted in favor of the hyperchromatic nuclei (May-Grünwald-Giemsa, 1,000×, oil immersion).

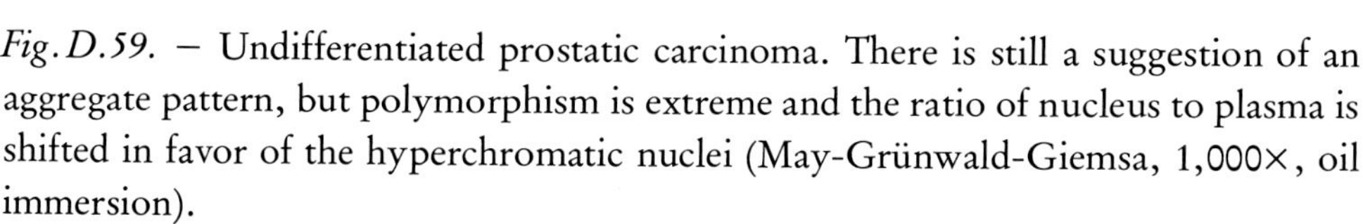

Fig.D.60. – Tumor cell in anaphase in an undifferentiated prostatic carcinoma. Tumor cells in mitosis are seldom found in prostatic carcinoma (May-Grünwald-Giemsa, 1,000×, oil immersion).

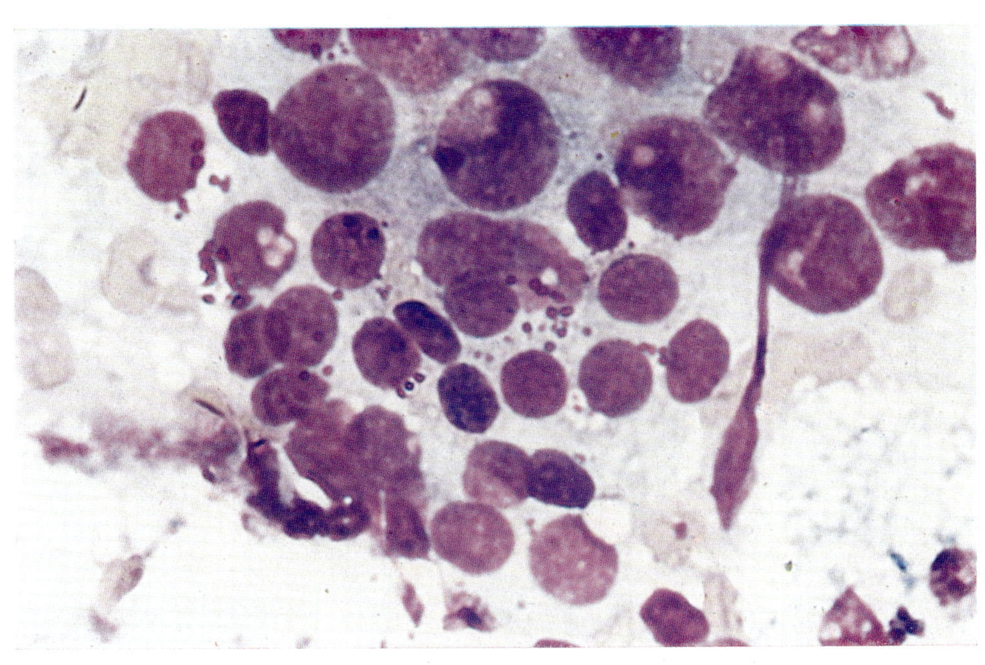

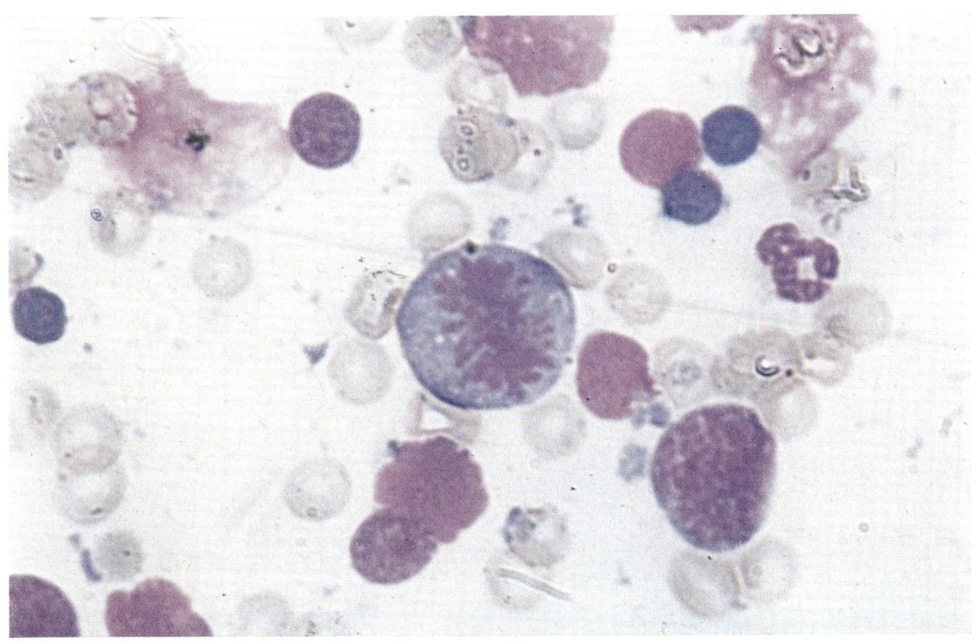

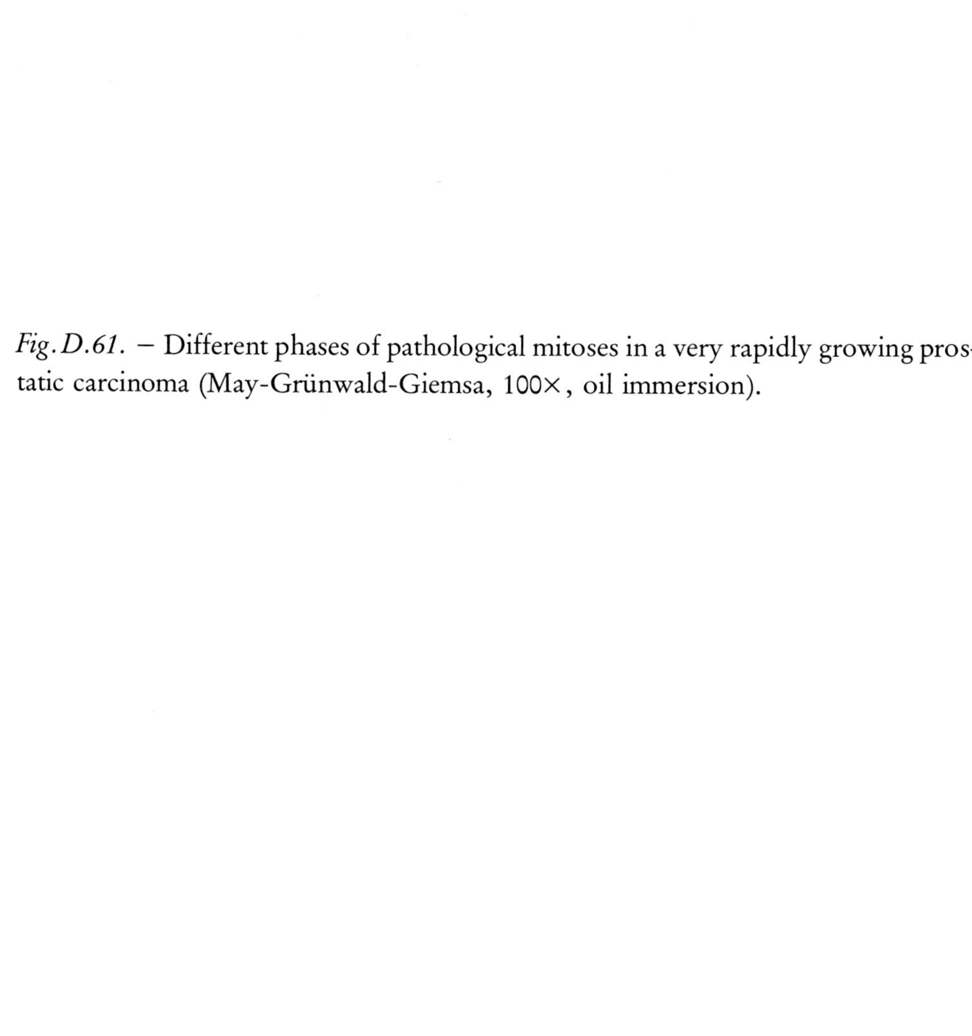

Fig. D.61. – Different phases of pathological mitoses in a very rapidly growing prostatic carcinoma (May-Grünwald-Giemsa, 100×, oil immersion).

Fig. D.62. – Marked dissociation of tumor cells. Most are naked, bizarre nuclei (May-Grünwald-Giemsa, 400×).

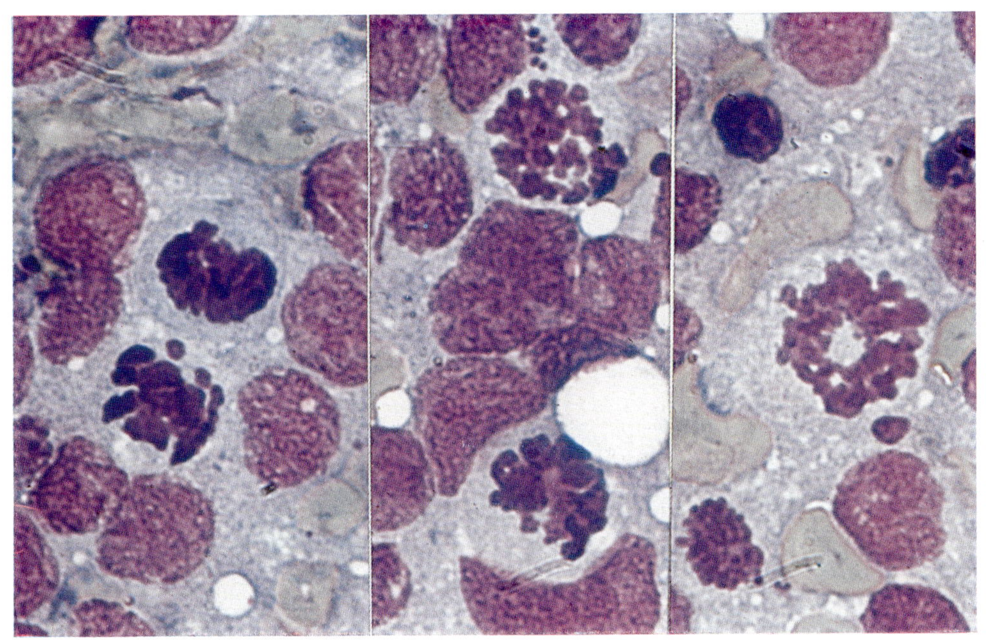

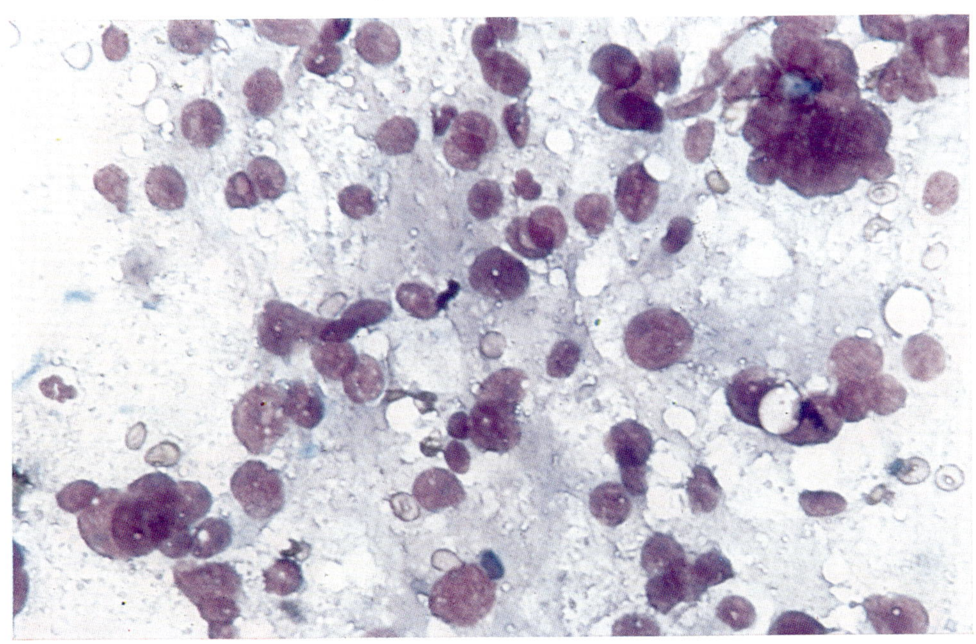

Fig. D.63. − Solitary, large tumor cell from an undifferentiated carcinoma. There is no cytoplasm to be seen. In the nucleoplasm at least six large, prominent nucleoli are visible in addition to three vacuoles that probably were caused by the air drying of the smear (May-Grünwald-Giemsa, 1,000×, oil immersion).

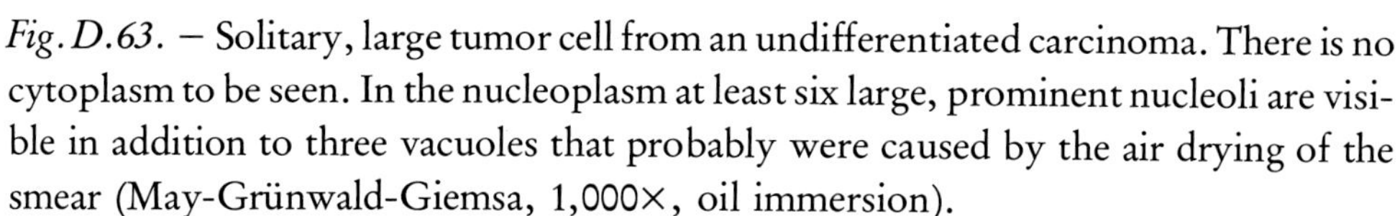

4. Effects of Hormone and Radiation Therapy on Nodular Hyperplasia and Carcinoma of the Prostate

Fig. D.64. − Histologic section of nodular hyperplasia of the prostate after six weeks treatment with estrogens (600 mg estradiol undecylat). The squamous epithelial metaplasia is plainly seen as well as inward growth and partial desquamation of epithelium into the lumen (semithin section, Movat silver stain, 400×).

92

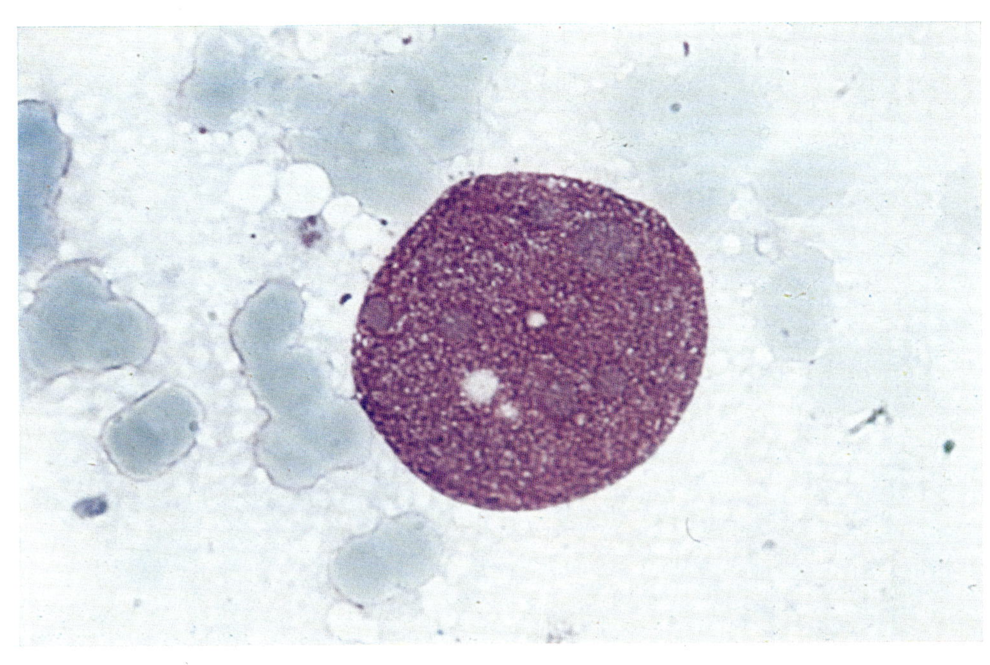

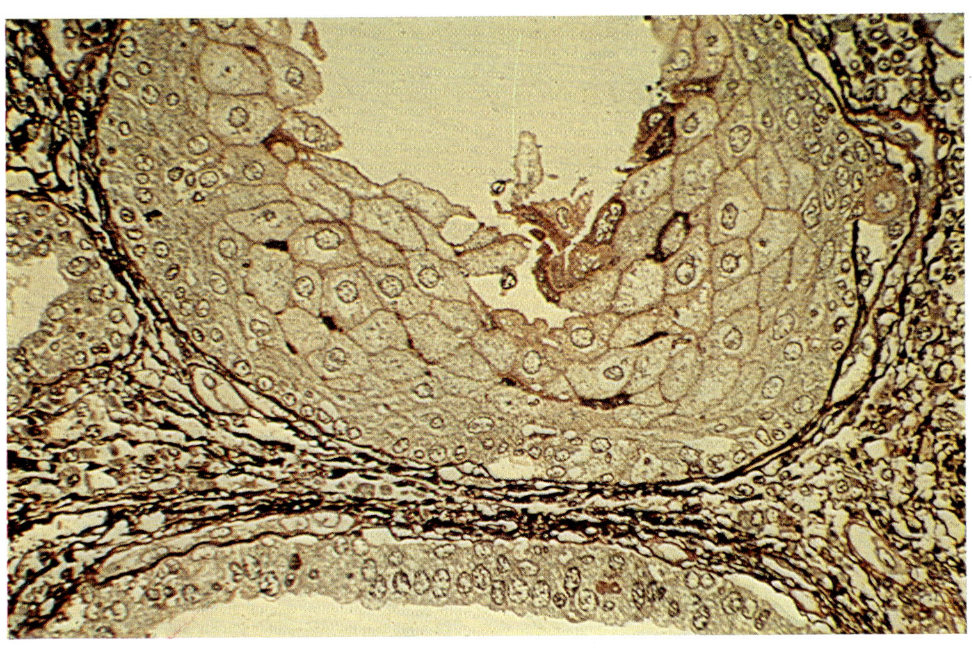

Fig. D.65. — Simultaneous biopsies of an estrogen-Treated case of nodular hyperplasia of the prostate. *Left,* the histologic preparation showing the typical pattern of squamous epithelium. *Right,* the cytologic smear in which there are metaplastic squamous epithelial cells which have arisen from the parabasal, intermediate, or superficial layers (left, HE, 250×; right, May-Grünwald-Giemsa, 250×).

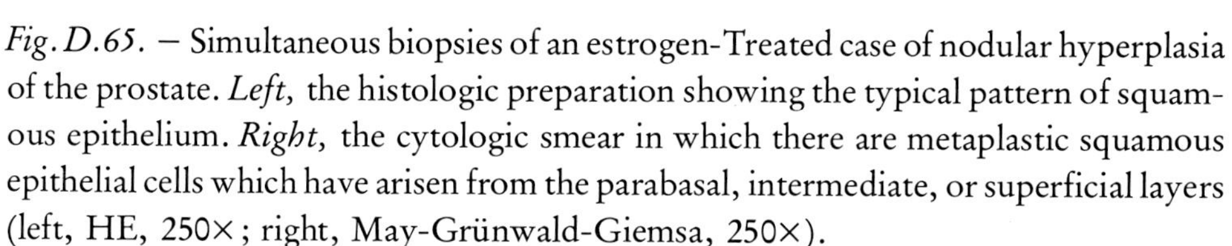

Fig. D.66. — Prostatic carcinoma six weeks after the start of estrogen therapy (total dose was 800 mg estradiol undecylat). The distinct vacuolization and thickening of the skeins of the chromatin framework of the carcinoma cells are typical signs of a good response to estrogen (May-Grünwald-Giemsa, 1,000×, oil immersion).

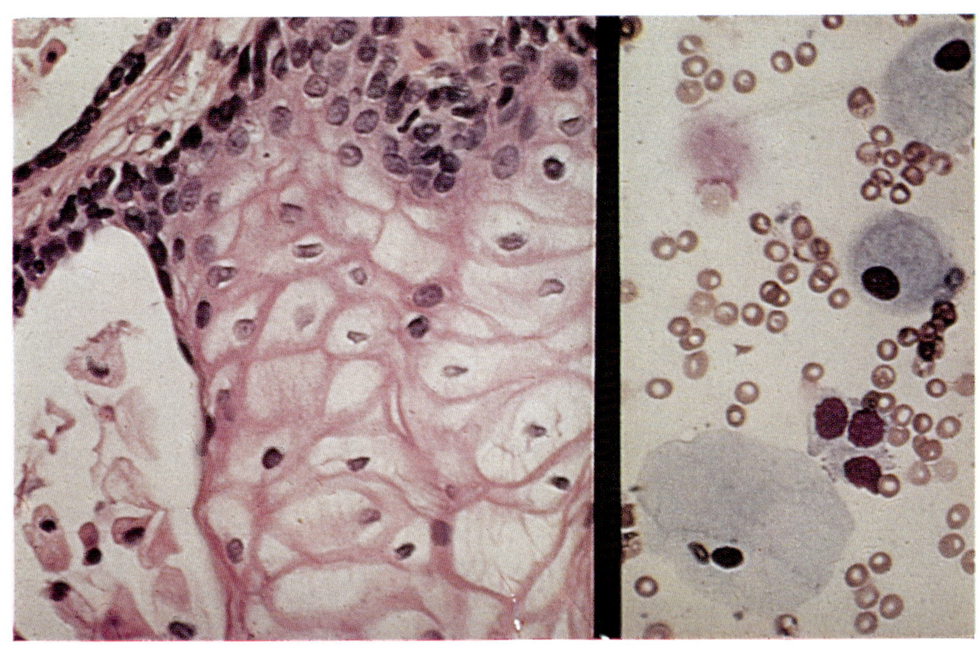

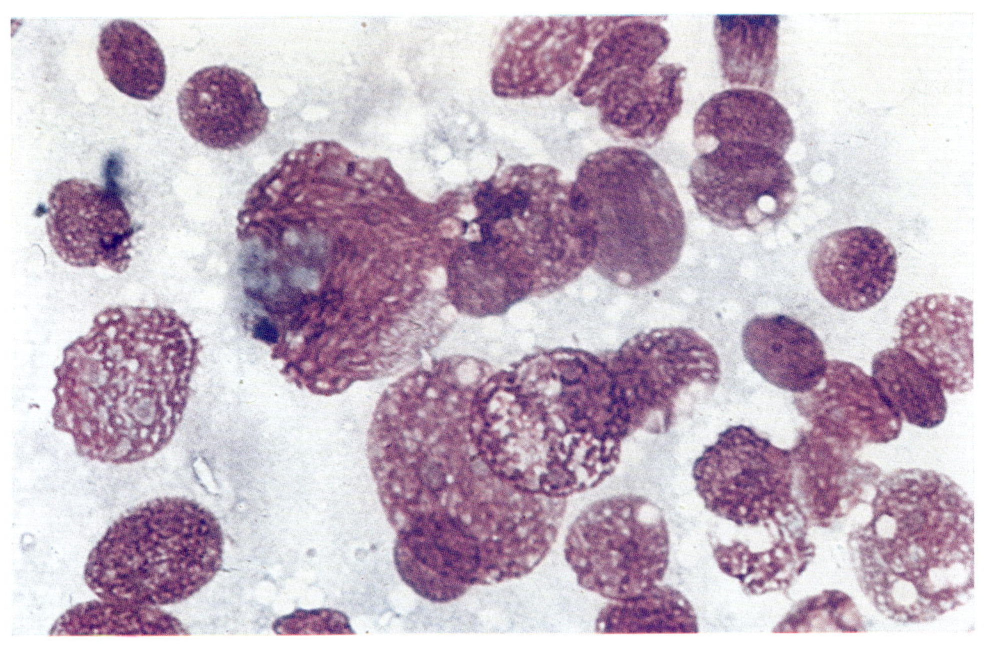

Fig.D.67. − Prostatic carcinoma. On the right are three large, metaplastic squamous epithelial cells coming from normal prostatic epithelium. On the left are carcinoma cells showing the loose arrangement of the interior of the nucleus and vacuolization. These findings indicate a good response of the carcinoma to the estrogen. In the middle of the upper border of the picture, the estrogenic effect can be detected in the degenerate, pyknotic nuclei (May-Grünwald-Giemsa, 1,000×, oil immersion).

Fig.D.68. − Moderately differentiated prostatic carcinoma showing estrogen effect. In the middle there is distinct squamous metaplasia of normal tissue. At the right border of the picture, there are aggregates of carcinoma cells showing estrogen-induced degenerative changes, although they are still recognizable as cancer cells. The changes in the carcinoma cells indicate a good response to estrogen therapy (May-Grünwald-Giemsa, 400×).

96

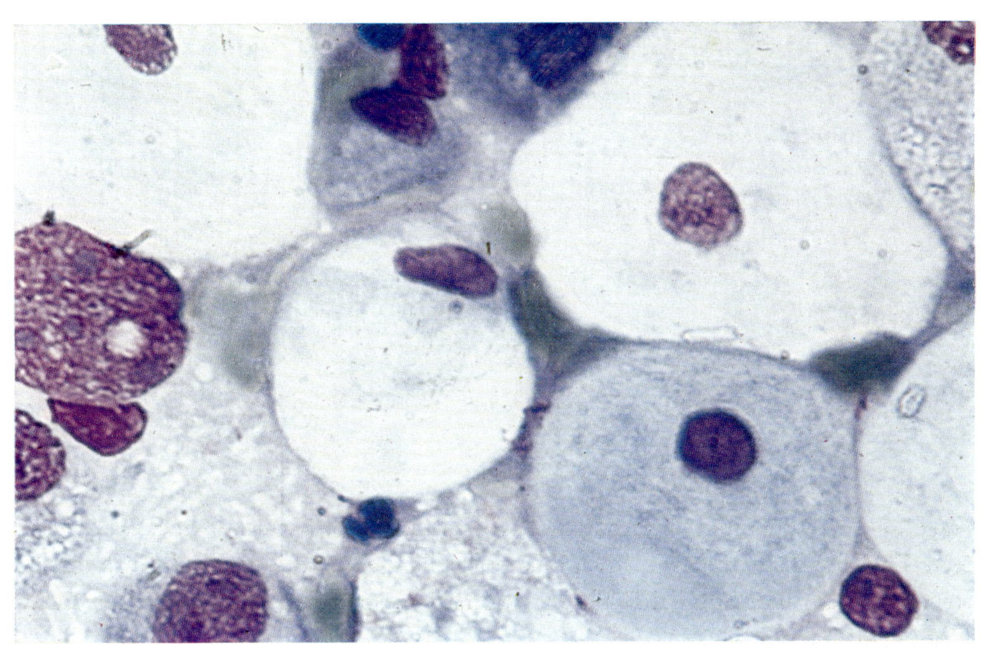

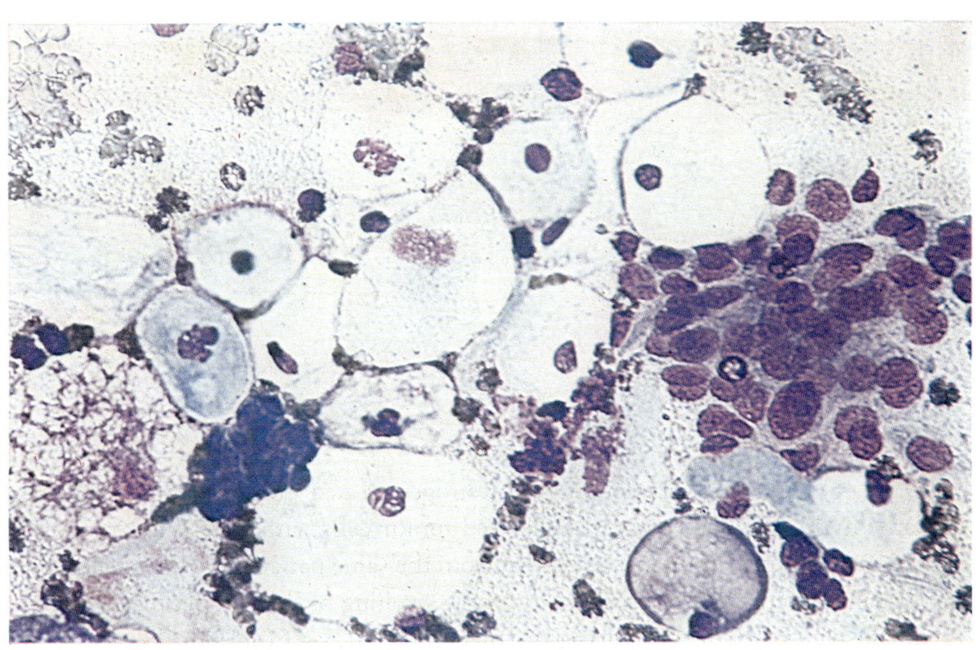

Fig. D.69. – Moderately differentiated prostatic carcinoma with distinct estrogen effect. Free-lying, metaplastic squamous epithelial cells are seen. The loose nuclear structure is an indication that the carcinoma is responding to the estrogen (May-Grünwald-Giemsa, 400×).

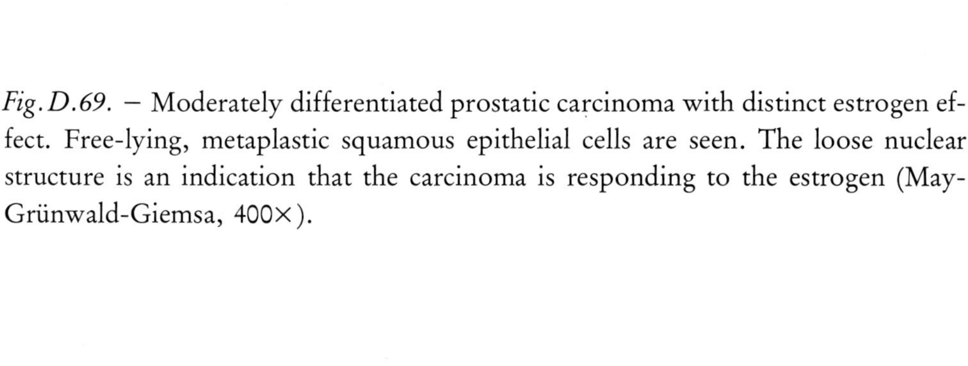

Fig. D.70. – *Left,* histologic section of an estrogen-treated prostatic carcinoma. There are large hydropically swollen, degenerated tumor cells with water-clear cytoplasm (HE, 330×). *Right,* simultaneous biopsy from the same patient showing chiefly pyknotic changes in the cancer cells and hydropic swelling of the cytoplasm. At the bottom of the picture, there is nonmalignant metaplasia (May-Grünwald-Giemsa, 400×).

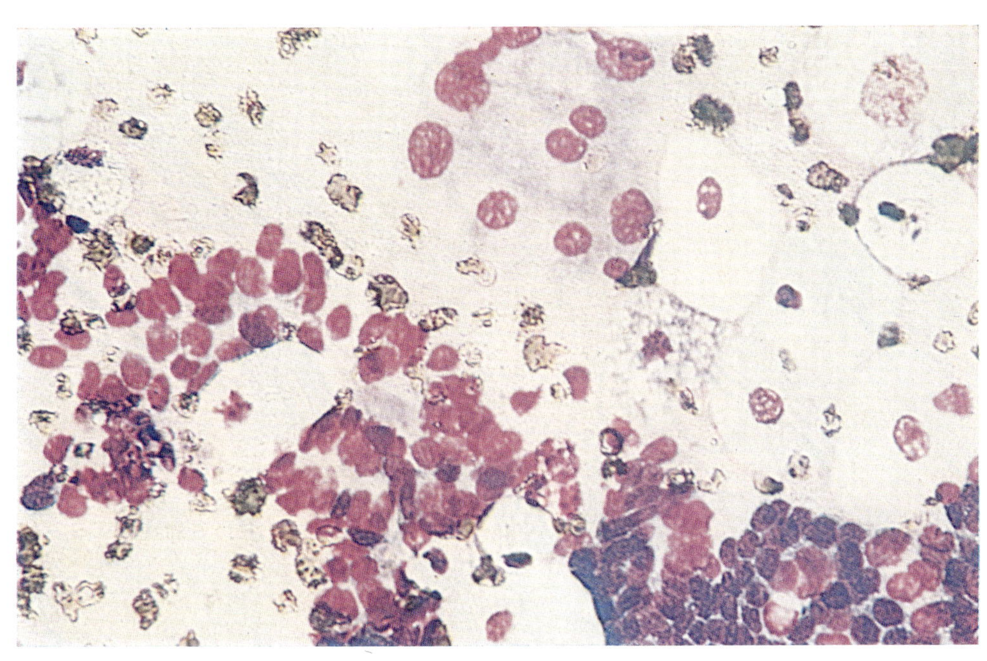

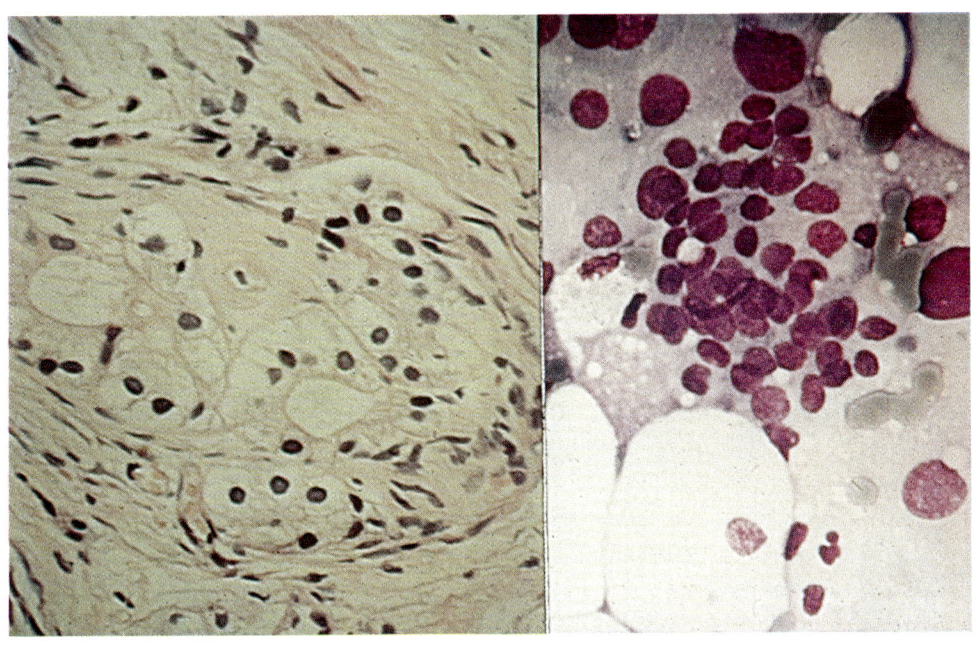

Fig.D.71. – Prostatic carcinoma showing a good response to estrogen. *Lower left,* squamous metplasia of epithelium; *upper left,* karyolysis of a carcinoma cell (May-Grünwald-Giemsa, 1,000×, oil immersion).

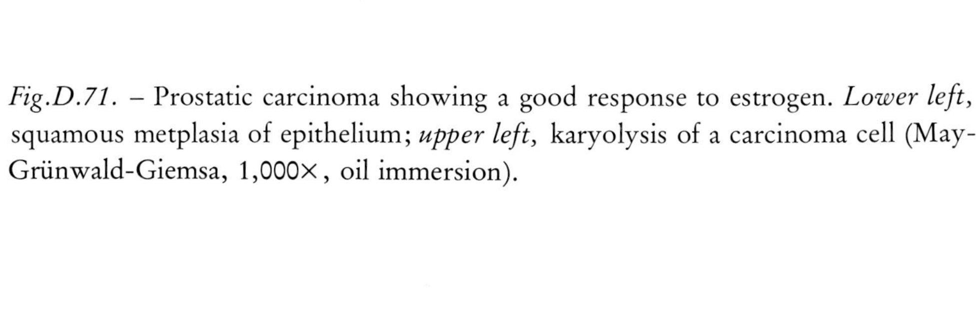

Fig.D.72. – Normal prostatic cells showing estrogen effect (400 mg estradiol undecylat). There is loosening of the sheet of cells with slight polymorphism and poly-chromasia, sporadic squamous metaplasia, and netlike thickening of the nucleoplasm (May-Grünwald-Giemsa, 250×).

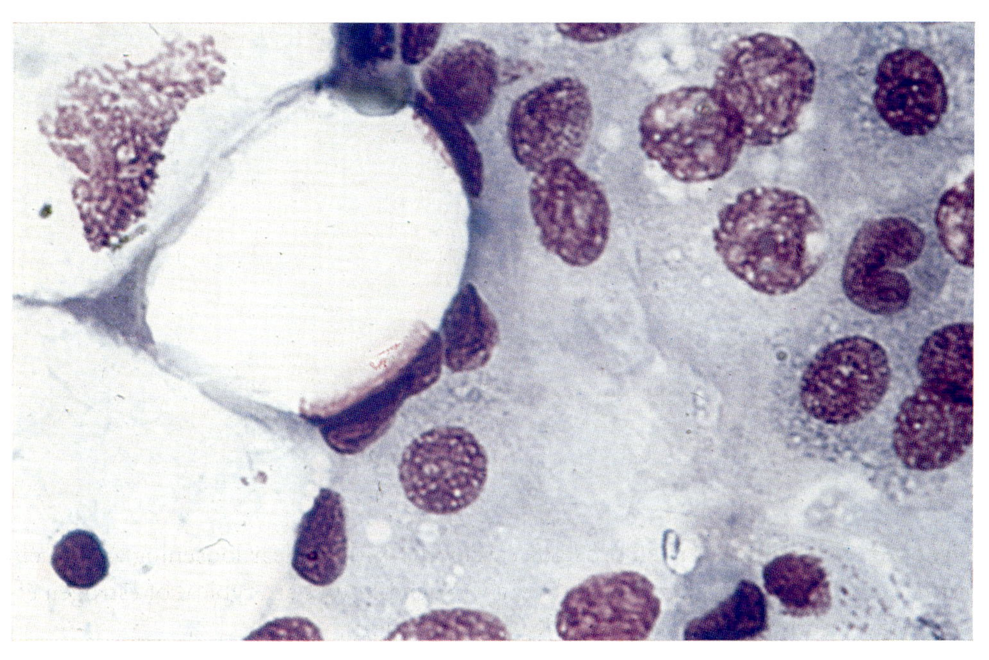

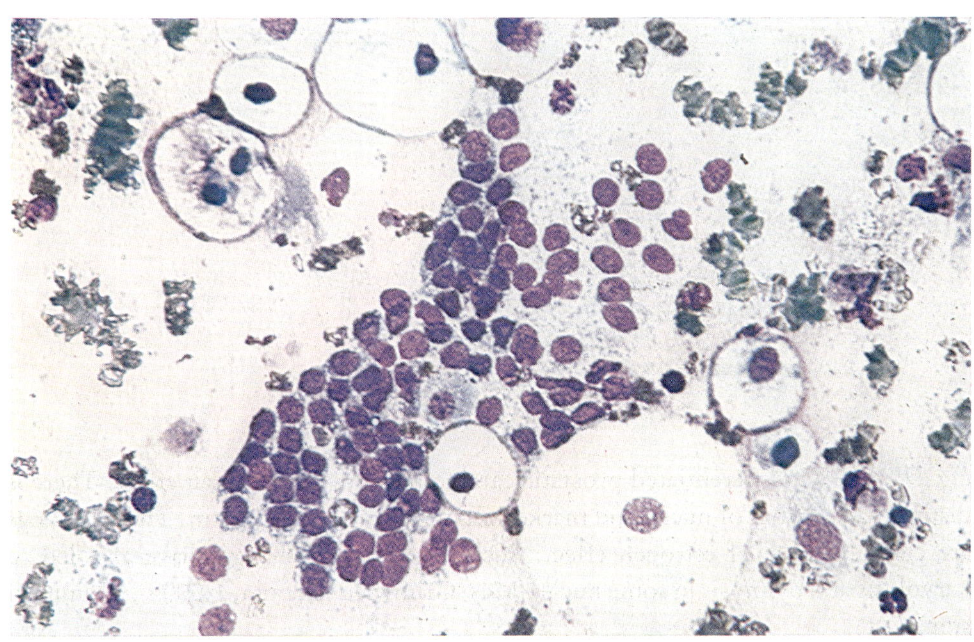

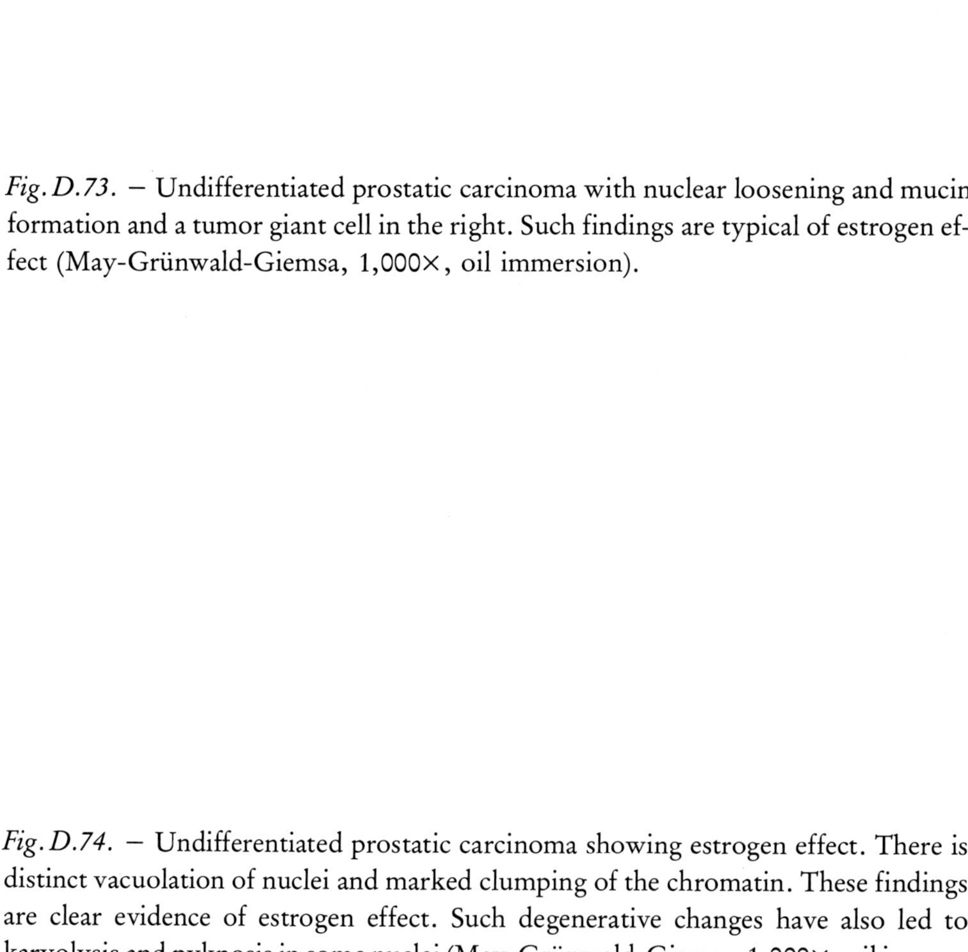

Fig. D.73. – Undifferentiated prostatic carcinoma with nuclear loosening and mucin formation and a tumor giant cell in the right. Such findings are typical of estrogen effect (May-Grünwald-Giemsa, 1,000×, oil immersion).

Fig. D.74. – Undifferentiated prostatic carcinoma showing estrogen effect. There is distinct vacuolation of nuclei and marked clumping of the chromatin. These findings are clear evidence of estrogen effect. Such degenerative changes have also led to karyolysis and pyknosis in some nuclei (May-Grünwald-Giemsa, 1,000×, oil immersion).

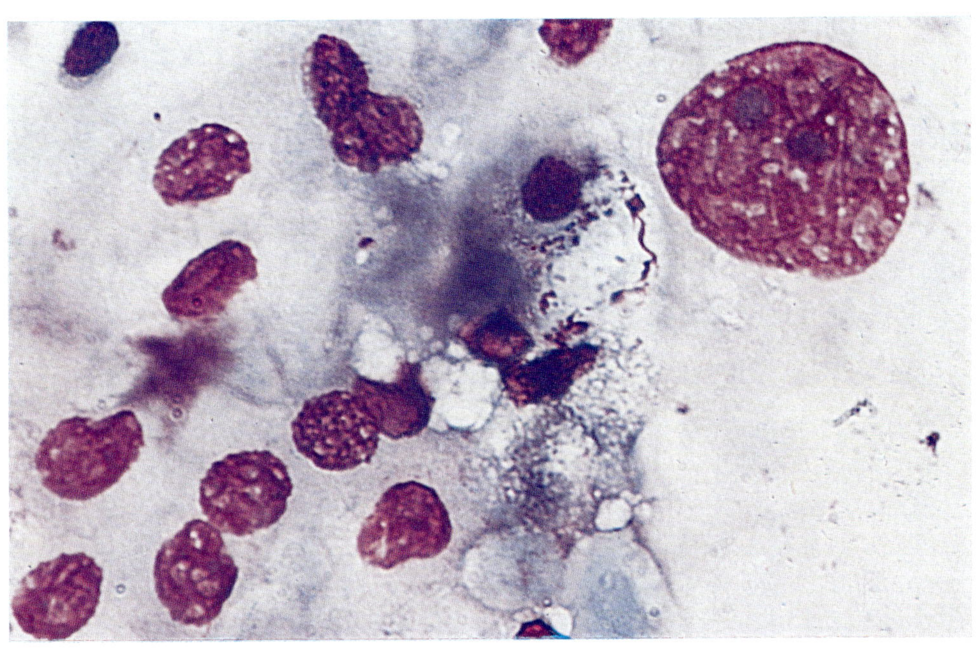

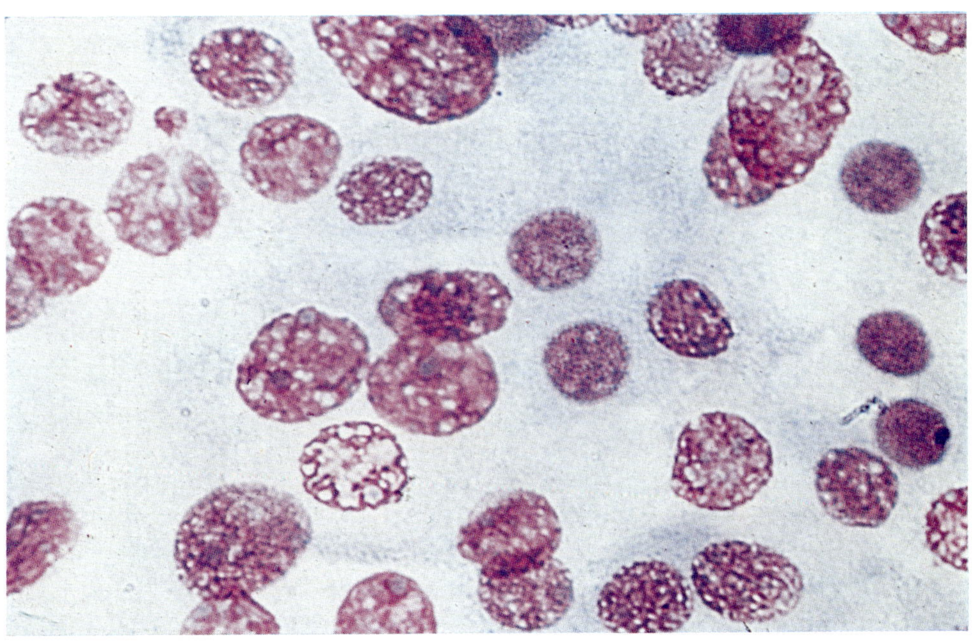

Fig. D.75. – Fluorescent microscopic preparation of a smear stained with acridine orange. It is from a prostatic carcinoma treated with estrogen. There are superficial layer cells in the middle with parabasal layer cells lying alongside. Above and to the left are two nuclei of carcinoma cells (acridine orange, 400×).

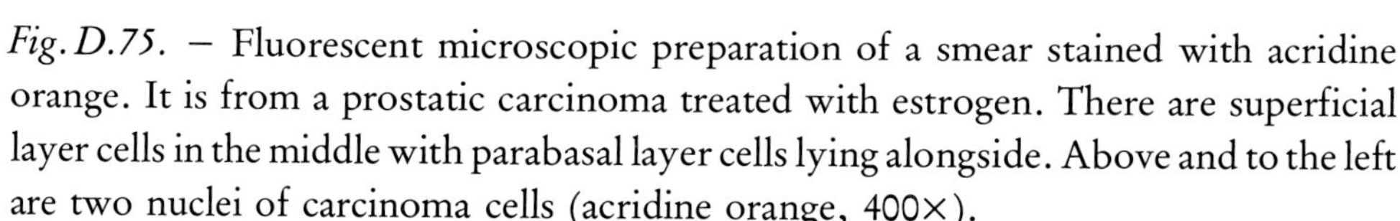

Fig. D.76. – "Glycogenic cells" in an estrogen-treated nodular prostatic hyperplasia. *Left,* metaplastic squamous epithelium stained with PAS. *Right,* another smear demonstrating enzymatic hydrolysis of the glycogen with amylase, which confirms the diagnosis. The glycogen has been degraded and therefore can no longer be stained with PAS (PAS, 250×).

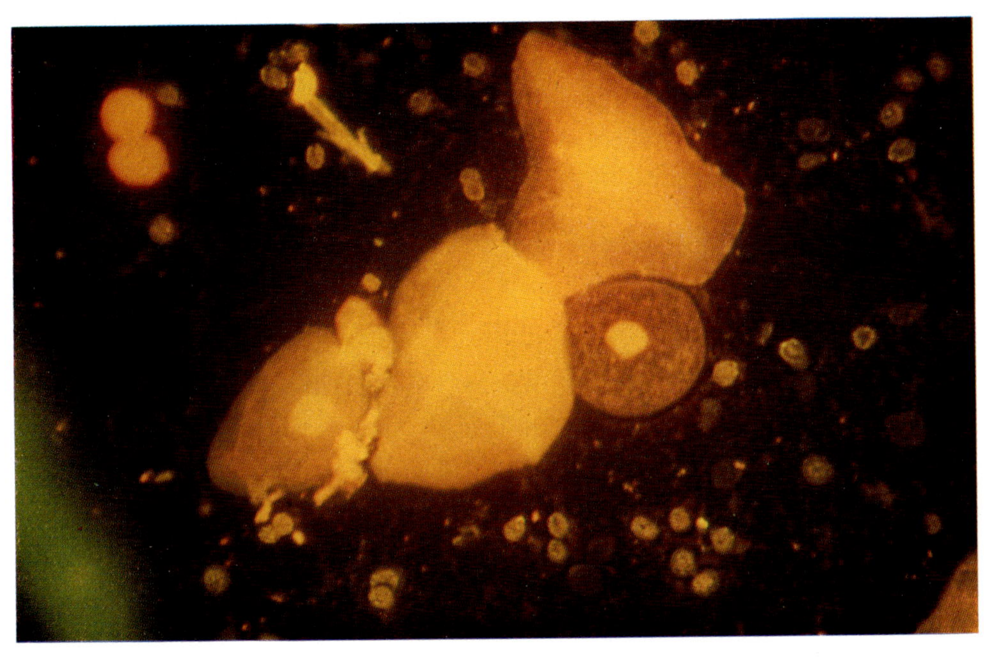

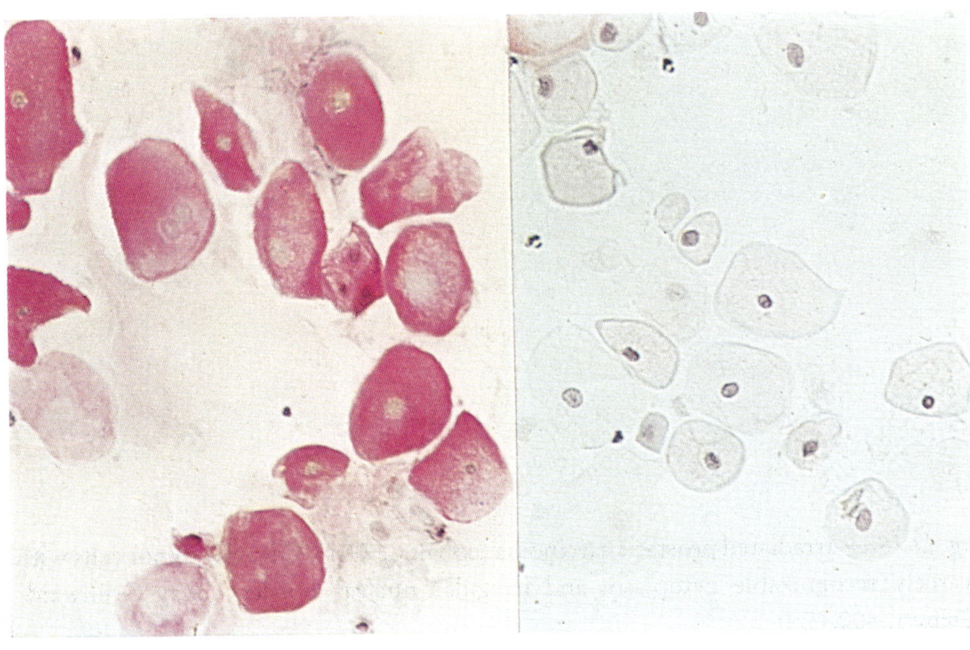

Fig. D.77. − Irradiated carcinoma of the prostate (cobalt 6,000 r). Typical large, confluent nuclei with irregular, vacuolar loosening of the nucleoplasm in some. Cell margins are absent and there are fingerlike excrescences on the irradiated nuclei (May-Grünwald-Giemsa, 400×).

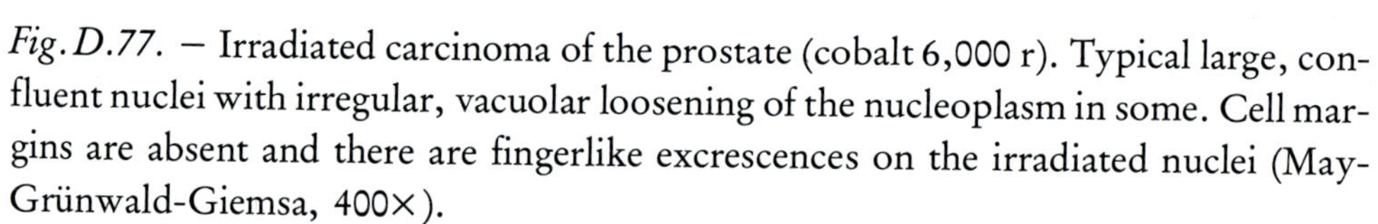

Fig. D.78. − Irradiated prostatic carcinoma (cobalt 6,000 r). Gigantic tumor cells with scarcely recognizable cytoplasm and irregular nuclear borders (May-Grünwald-Giemsa, 400×).

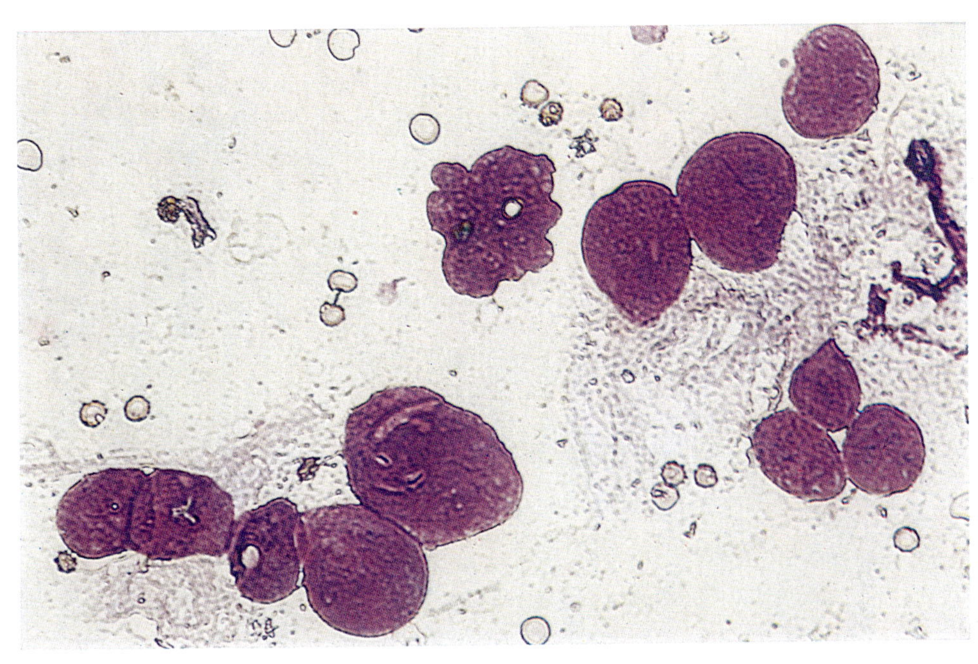

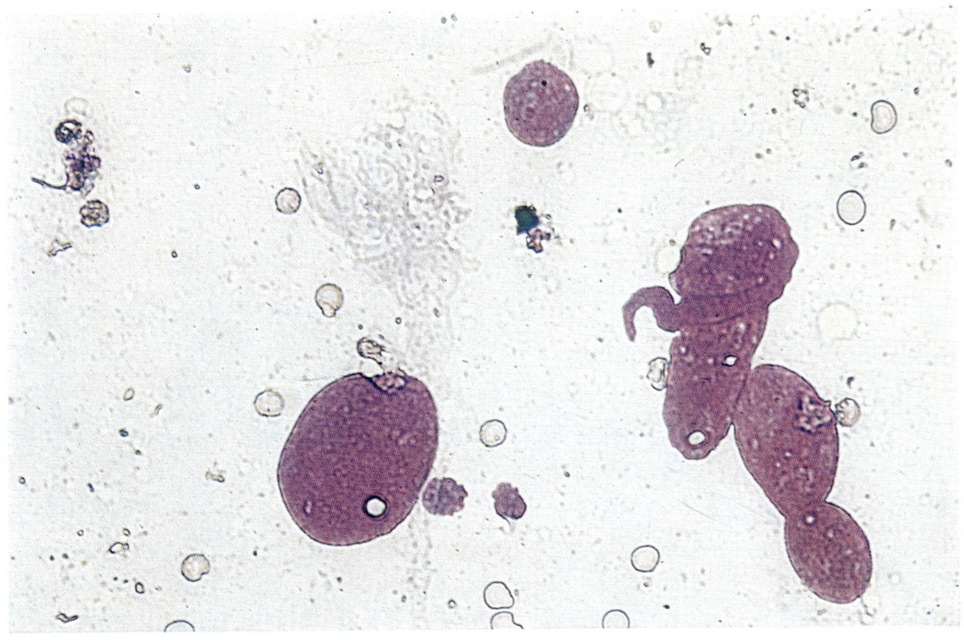

Fig. D.79. – Prostatic carcinoma irradiated with cobalt, showing confluent nuclei and bizarre excrescences in some (May-Grünwald-Giemsa, 400×).

5. Cells Concomitantly Aspirated from Neighboring Organs

a) Seminal Vesicle

Fig. D.80. – Histologic preparation of normal seminal vesicle from a 29-year-old man. There is considerable polymorphism and polychromasia of the nuclei of the lining epithelium. Many nuclei at the base of the folds of the mucous membrane are large and have a loosely arranged nuclear structure. At the top of the folds, there is less difference in nuclear size and the chromatin structure is denser (HE, 1,250×, oil immersion).

108

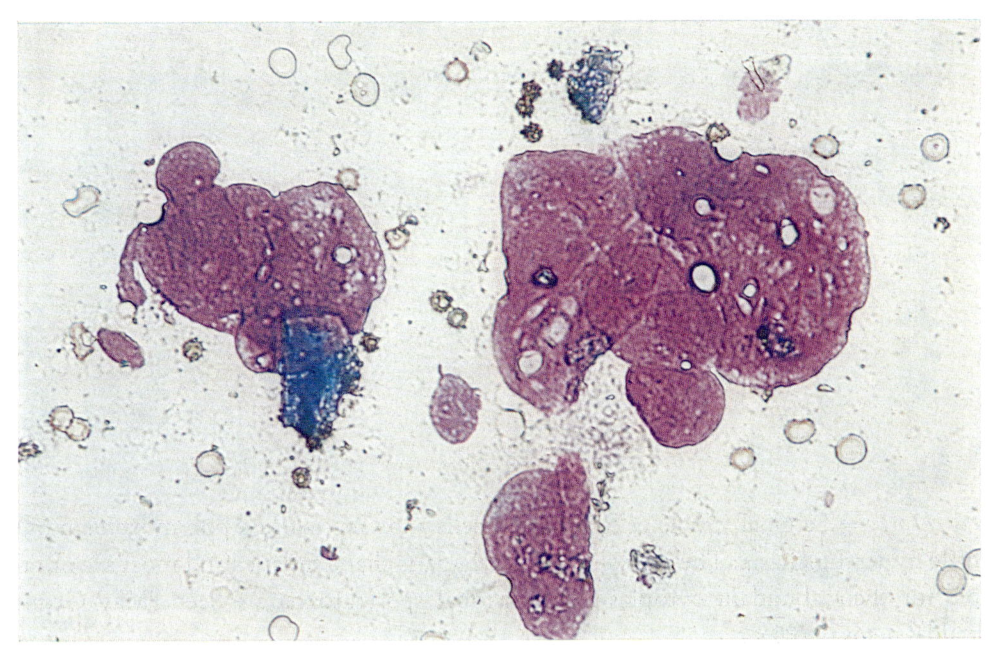

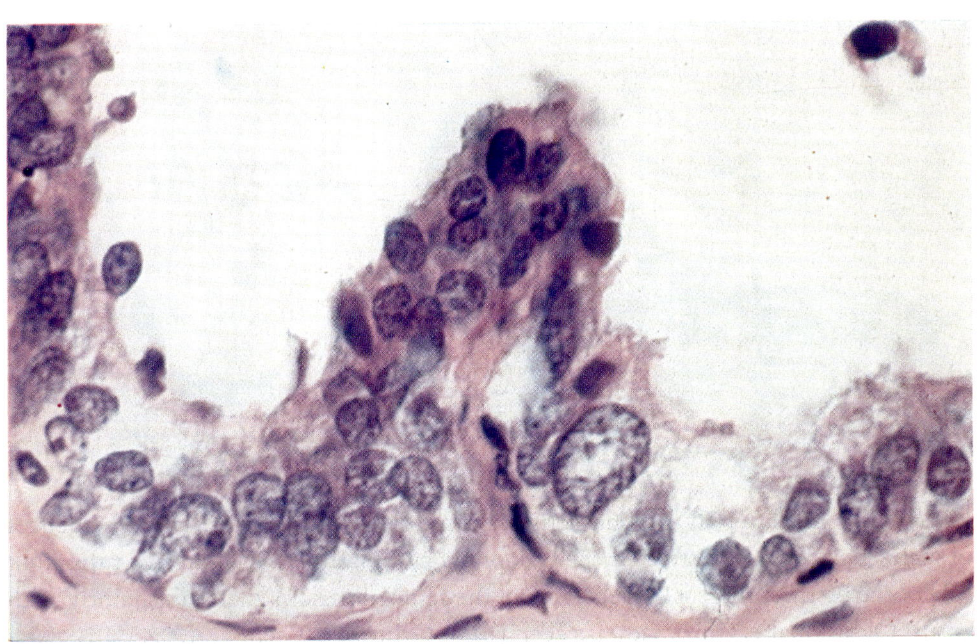

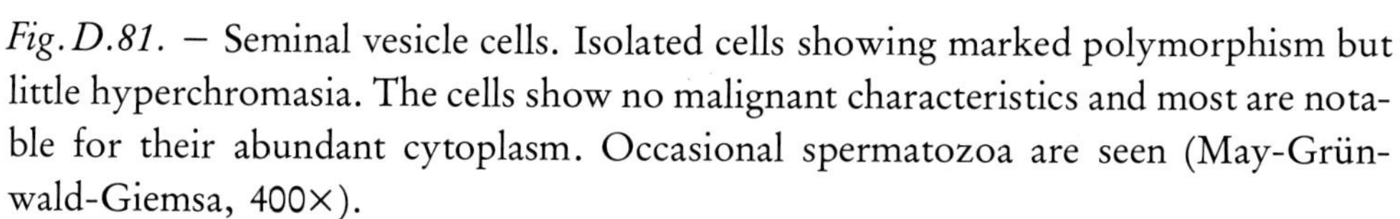

Fig. D.81. – Seminal vesicle cells. Isolated cells showing marked polymorphism but little hyperchromasia. The cells show no malignant characteristics and most are notable for their abundant cytoplasm. Occasional spermatozoa are seen (May-Grünwald-Giemsa, 400×).

Fig. D.82. – Typical polymorphic cells of the seminal vesicles. There are no evidences of malignancy and in some cells the basophilic cytoplasm is vacuolated. At the right side of the picture, there is secretion from the seminal vesicles that stains faintly with eosin. Occasional erythrocytes are seen (May-Grünwald-Giemsa, 400×).

110

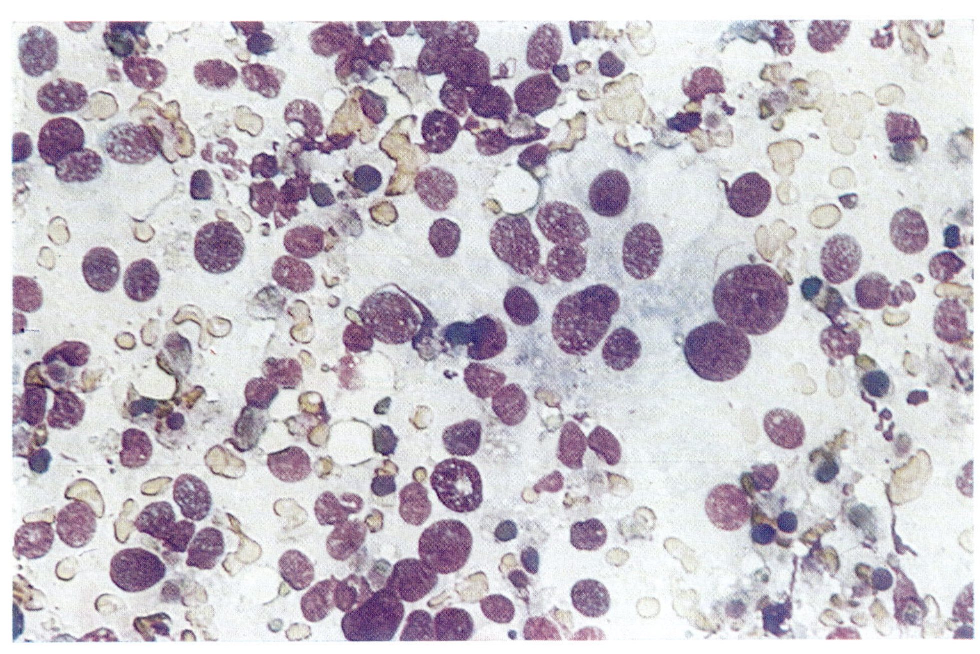

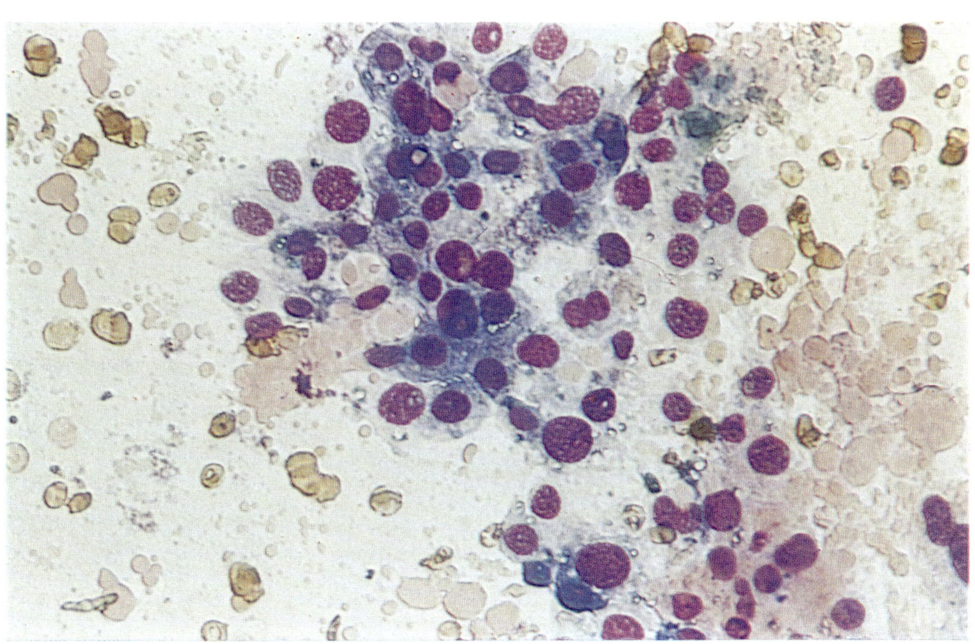

Fig.D.83. – Sheet of seminal vesicle cells partially overlapped. The large polymorphic cells are remarkable and reminiscent of rhabdomyosarcoma. Such large nuclei do not occur in the prostate itself. Distinct cytoplasmic borders and secretion are present in the smear, but there are no evidences of malignancy (May-Grünwald-Giemsa, 400×).

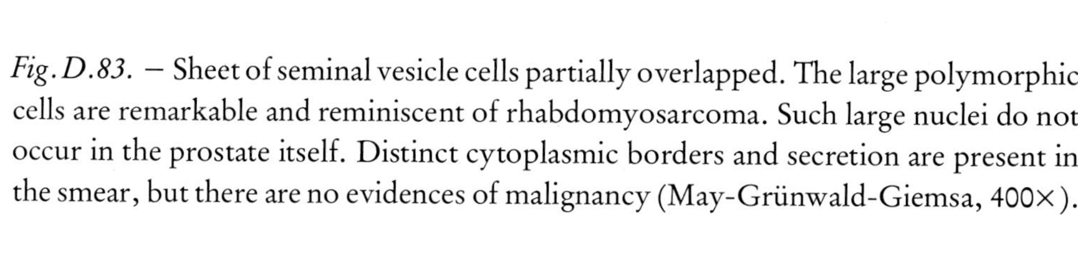

Fig.D.84. – Four seminal vesicle cells lie in the upper part of the picture and beneath them some prostatic cells. The marked difference between them is clear. The seminal vesicle cells have abundant cytoplasm, and their nuclei show no malignant characteristics except for polymorphism (May-Grünwald-Giemsa, 400×).

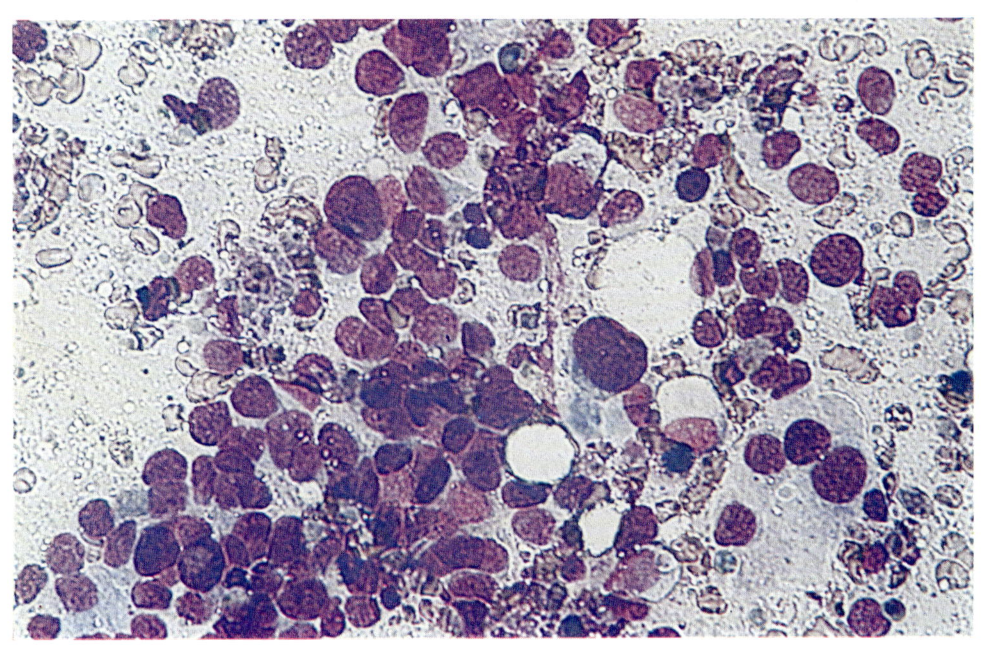

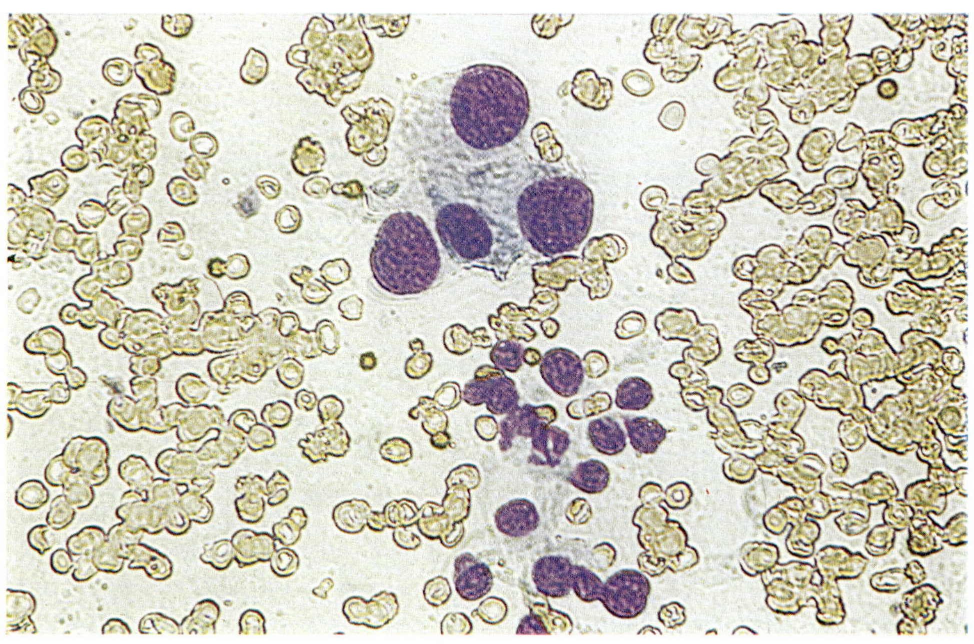

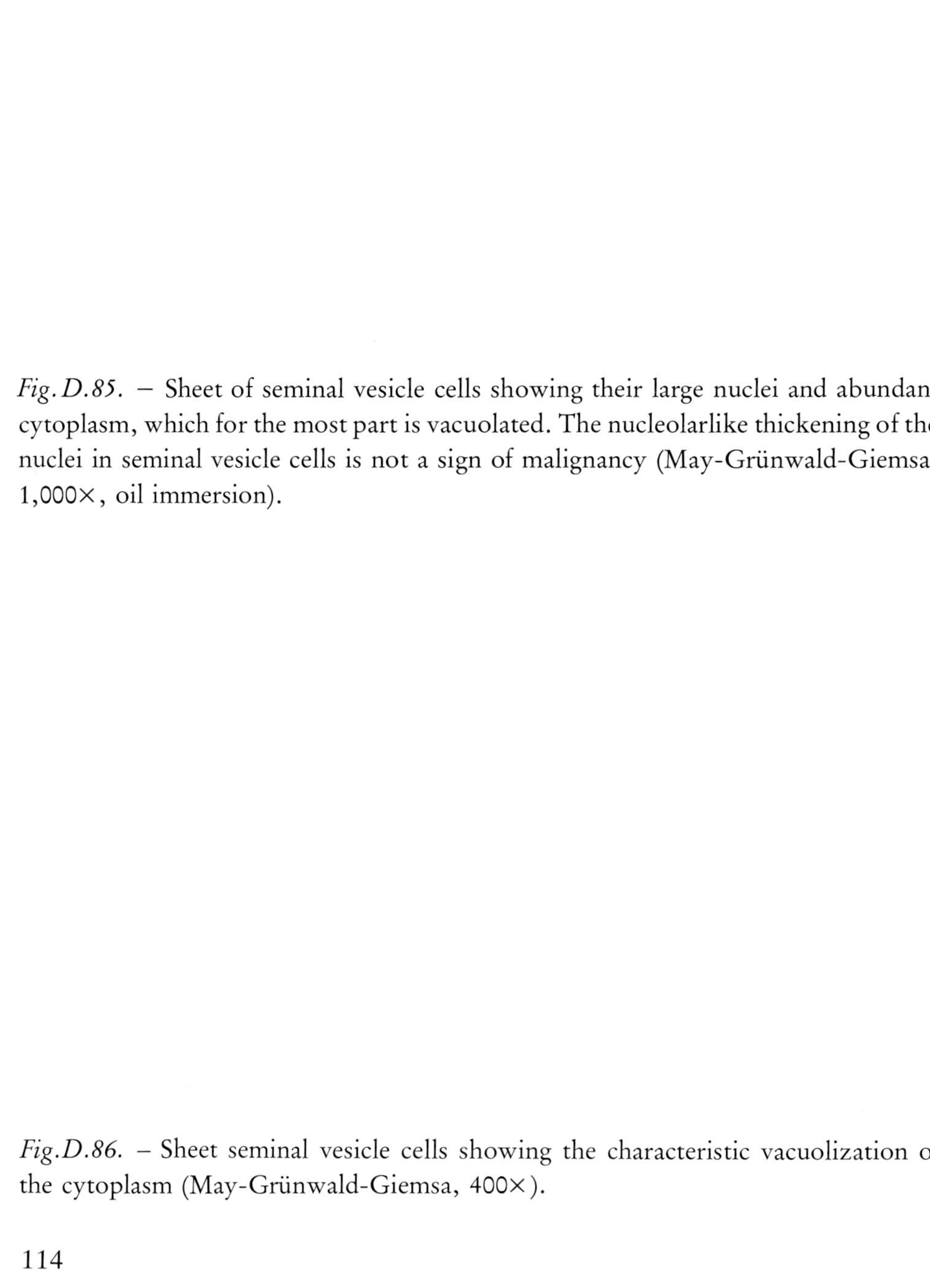

Fig.D.85. – Sheet of seminal vesicle cells showing their large nuclei and abundant cytoplasm, which for the most part is vacuolated. The nucleolarlike thickening of the nuclei in seminal vesicle cells is not a sign of malignancy (May-Grünwald-Giemsa, 1,000×, oil immersion).

Fig.D.86. – Sheet seminal vesicle cells showing the characteristic vacuolization of the cytoplasm (May-Grünwald-Giemsa, 400×).

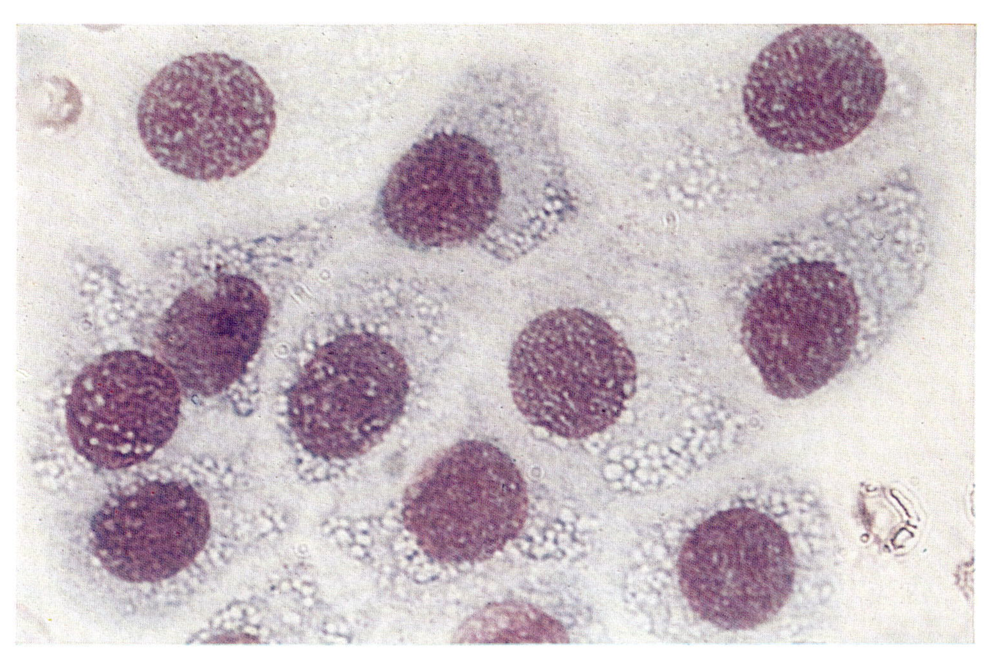

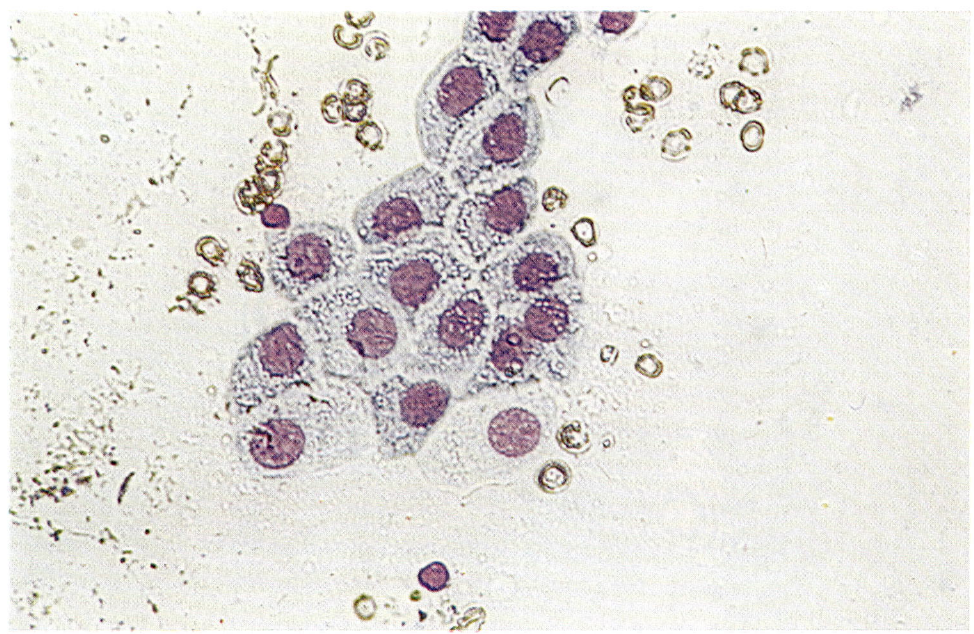

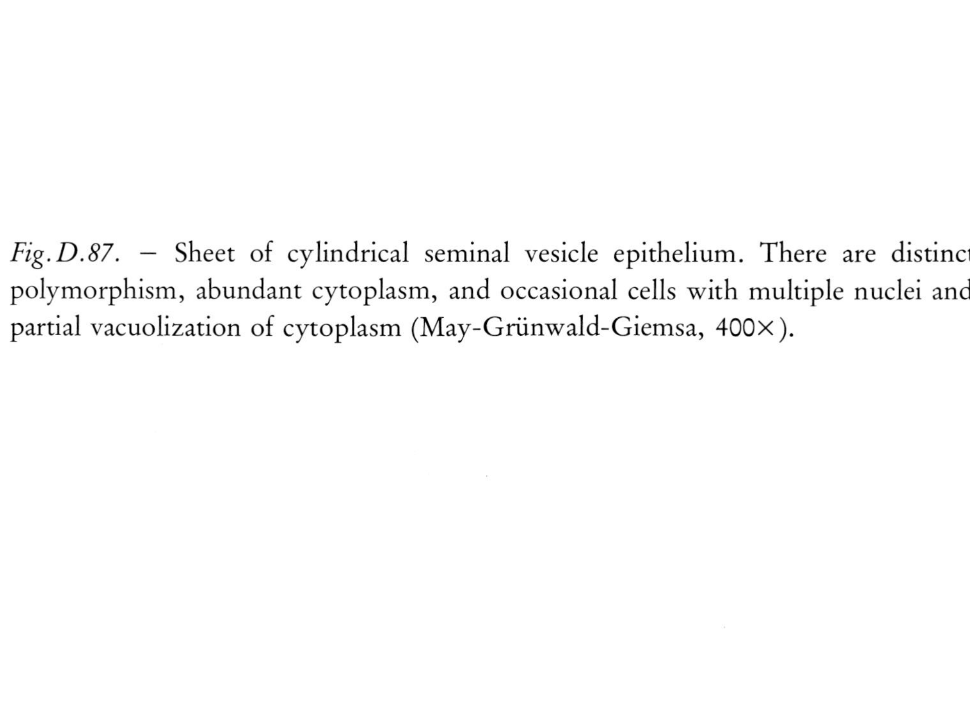

Fig. D.87. – Sheet of cylindrical seminal vesicle epithelium. There are distinct polymorphism, abundant cytoplasm, and occasional cells with multiple nuclei and partial vacuolization of cytoplasm (May-Grünwald-Giemsa, 400×).

Fig. D.88. – Histologic preparation of the cranial portion of the normal ductus deferens of a 29-year-old man. There is a relatively uniform, double layer of epithelium with small, round nuclei in the basal layer of the mucosa and a superficial layer of ciliated cylindrical cells, many of which are vacuolated (HE, 1,250×, oil immersion).

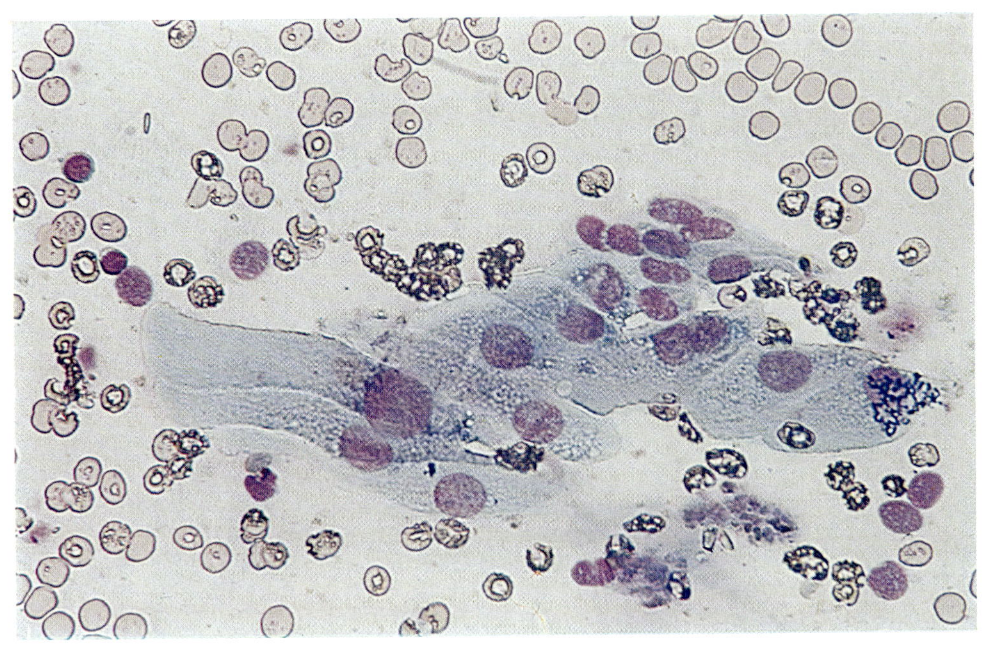

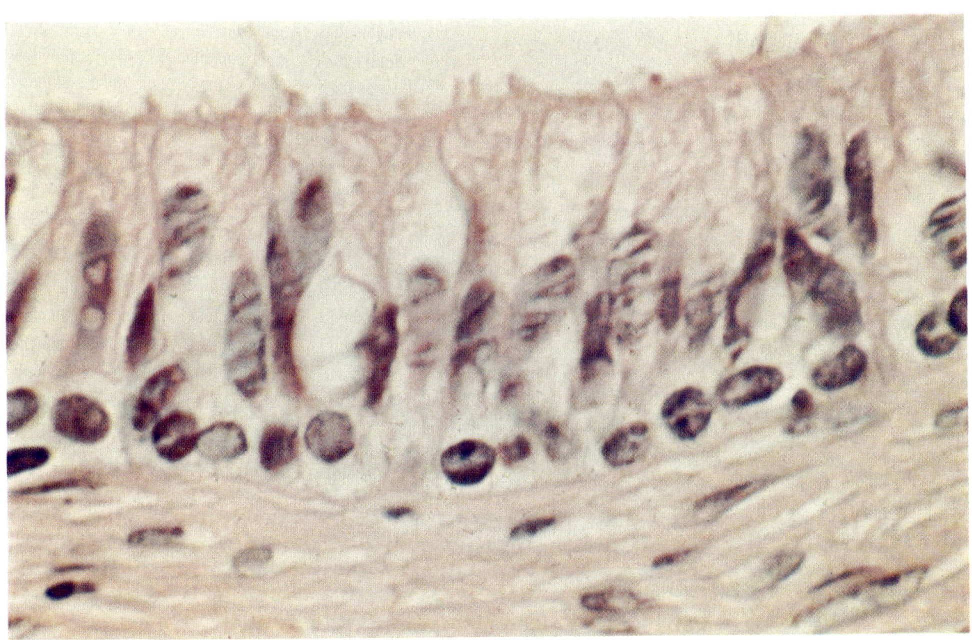

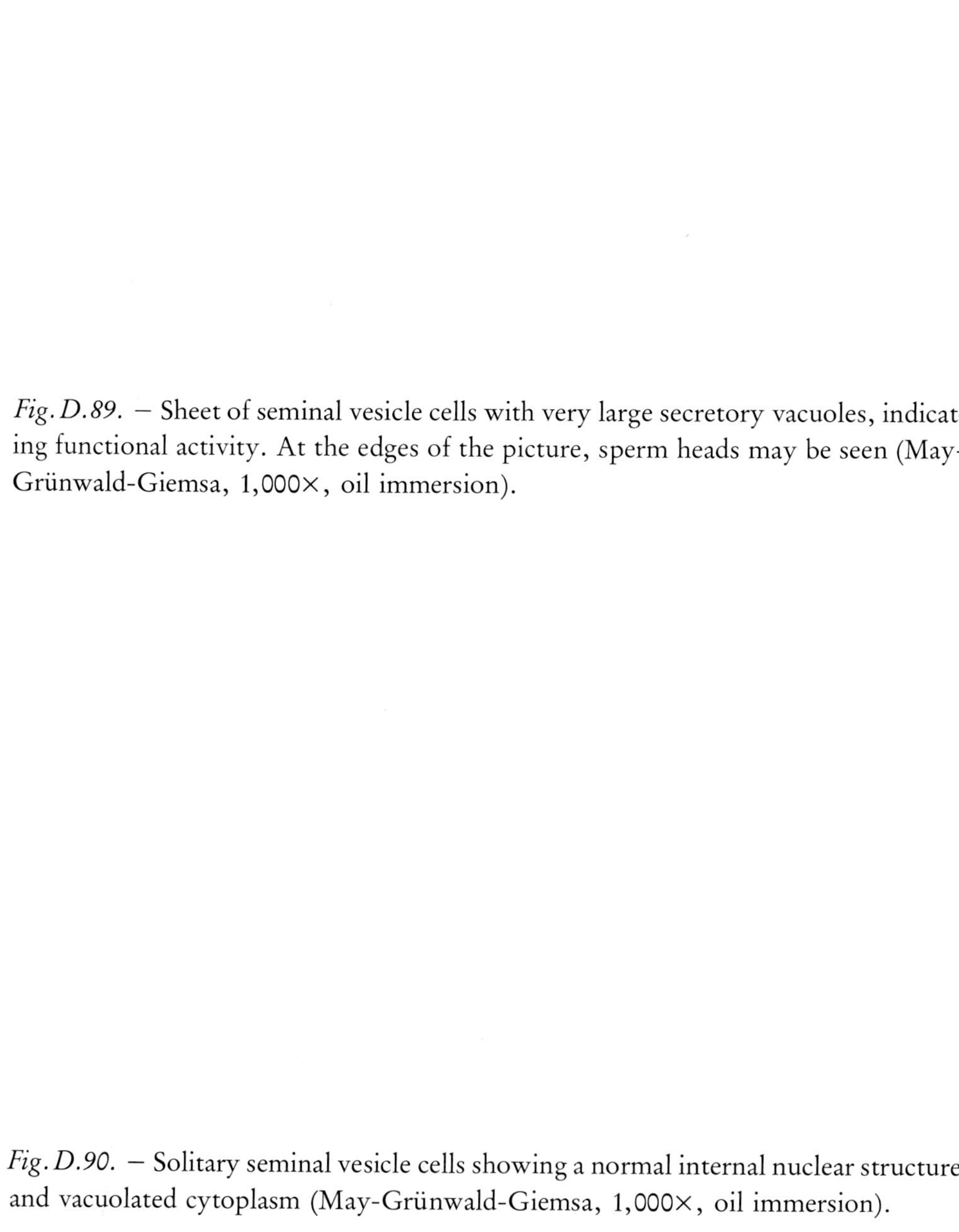

Fig. D.89. – Sheet of seminal vesicle cells with very large secretory vacuoles, indicating functional activity. At the edges of the picture, sperm heads may be seen (May-Grünwald-Giemsa, 1,000×, oil immersion).

Fig. D.90. – Solitary seminal vesicle cells showing a normal internal nuclear structure and vacuolated cytoplasm (May-Grünwald-Giemsa, 1,000×, oil immersion).

118

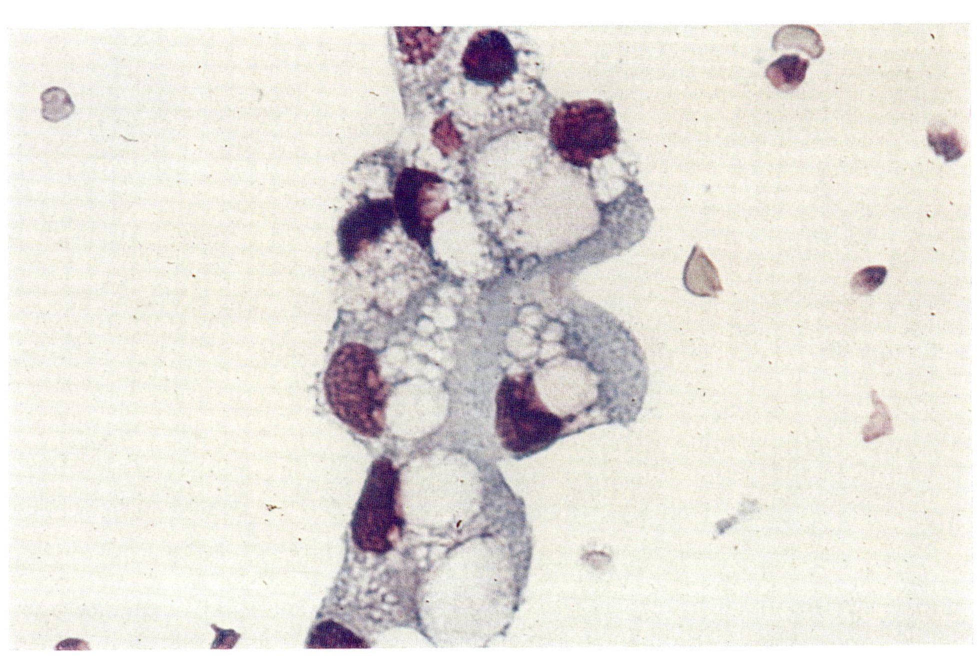

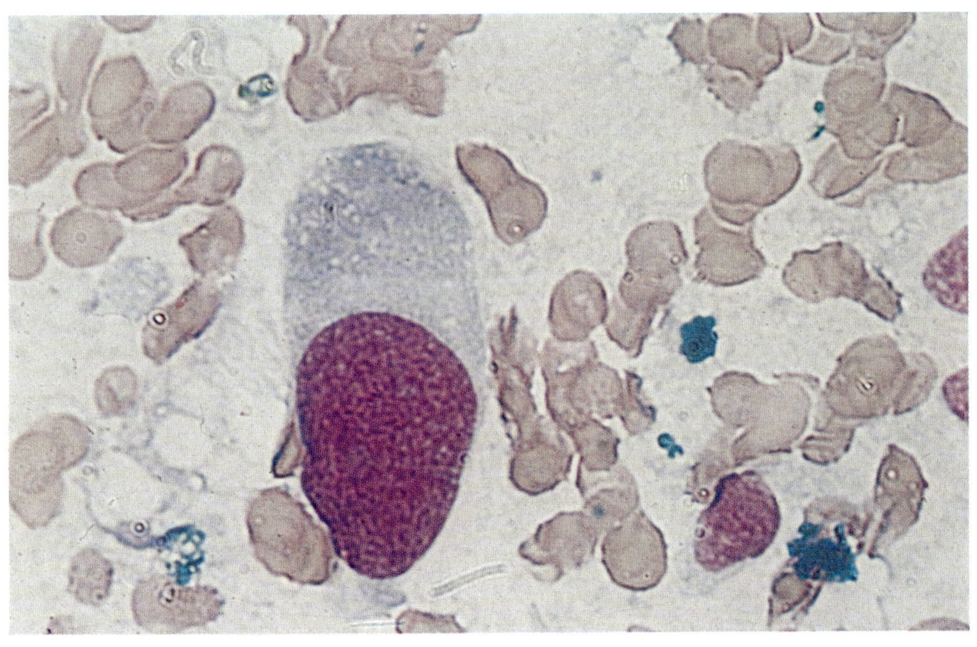

Fig. D.91. – Sheet of prostatic cells above, lying next to seminal vesicle epithelium below, which are distinguished by their difference in size and their vacuolated cytoplasm. Aggregates of erythrocytes surround them (May-Grünwald-Giemsa, 400×).

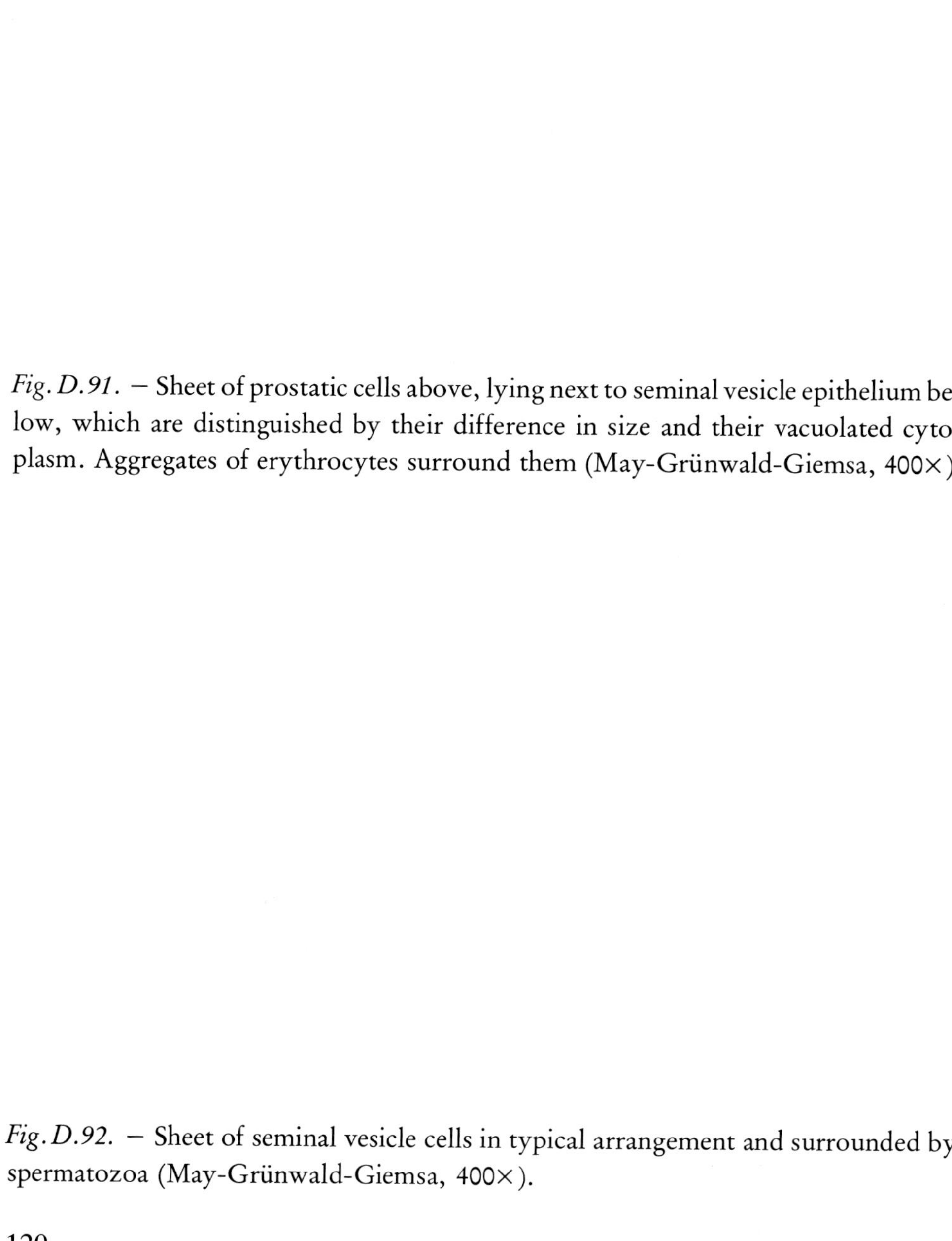

Fig. D.92. – Sheet of seminal vesicle cells in typical arrangement and surrounded by spermatozoa (May-Grünwald-Giemsa, 400×).

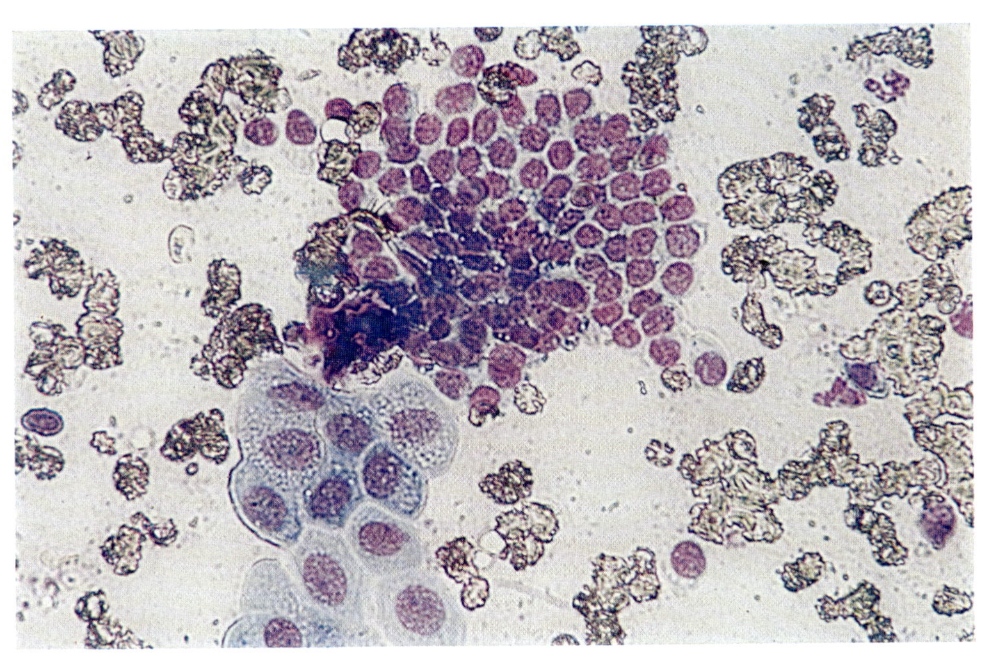

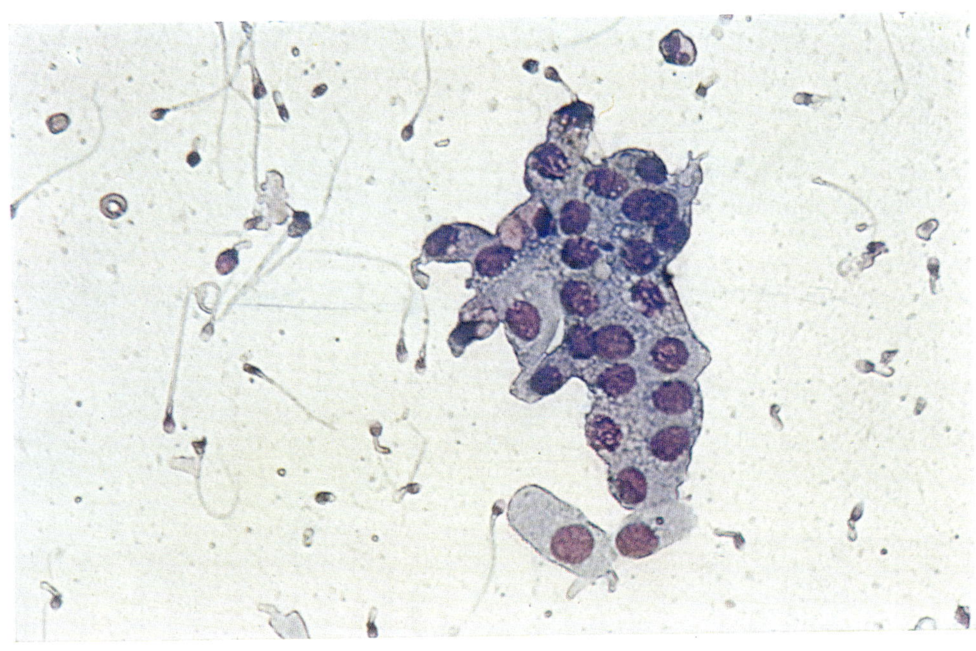

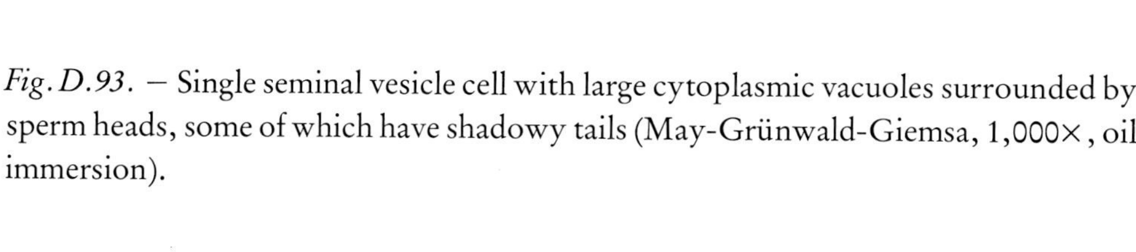

Fig. D.93. – Single seminal vesicle cell with large cytoplasmic vacuoles surrounded by sperm heads, some of which have shadowy tails (May-Grünwald-Giemsa, 1,000×, oil immersion).

Fig. D.94. – Sheet of seminal vesicle cells with moderately polymorphic nuclei (May-Grünwald-Giemsa, 1,000×, oil immersion).

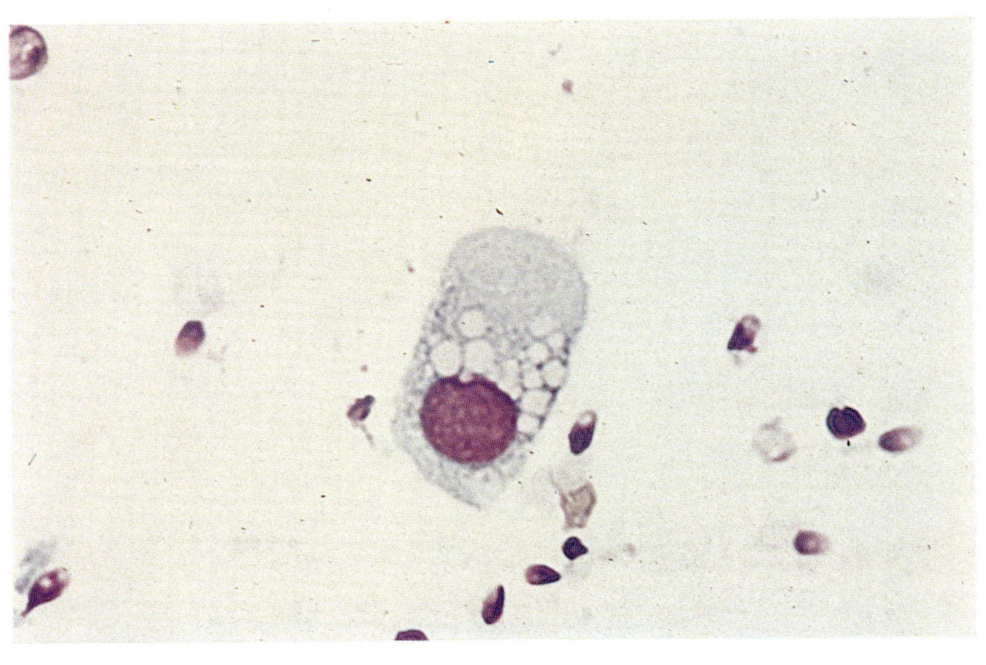

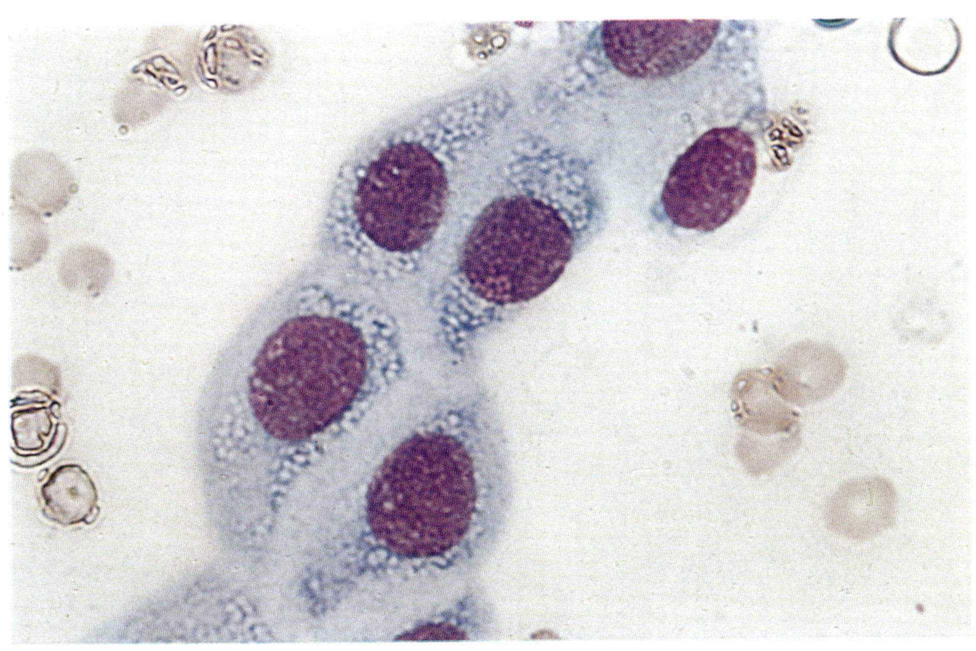

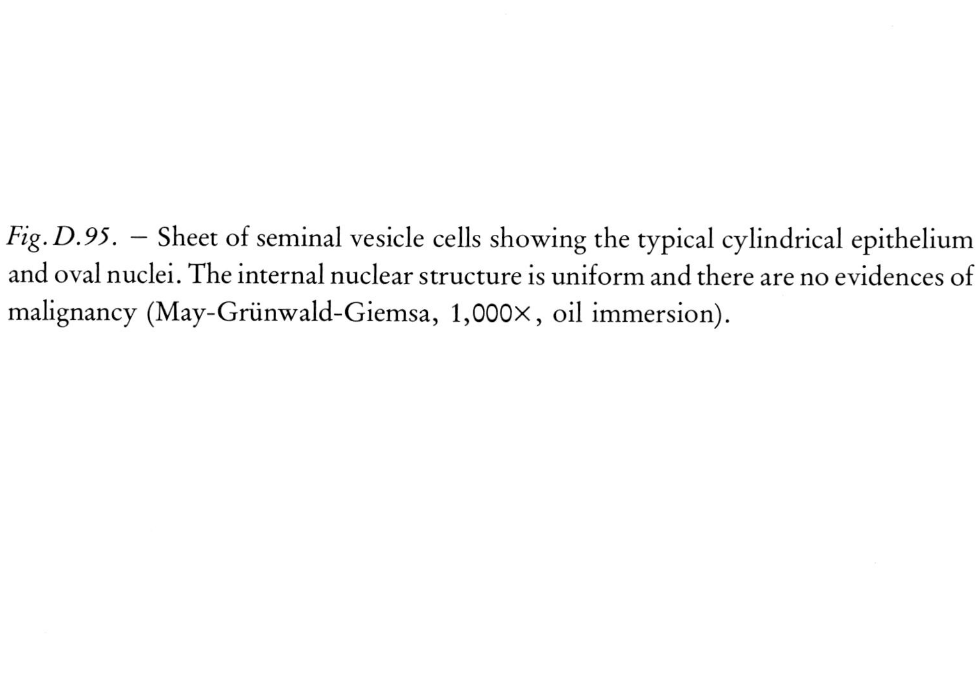

Fig. D.95. – Sheet of seminal vesicle cells showing the typical cylindrical epithelium and oval nuclei. The internal nuclear structure is uniform and there are no evidences of malignancy (May-Grünwald-Giemsa, 1,000×, oil immersion).

Fig. D.96. – Sheet from the seminal vesicle. There are cylindrical epithelial cells with abundant cytoplasm and somewhat marked nuclear polymorphism and poly-chromasia but no signs of malignancy (May-Grünwald-Giemsa, 400×).

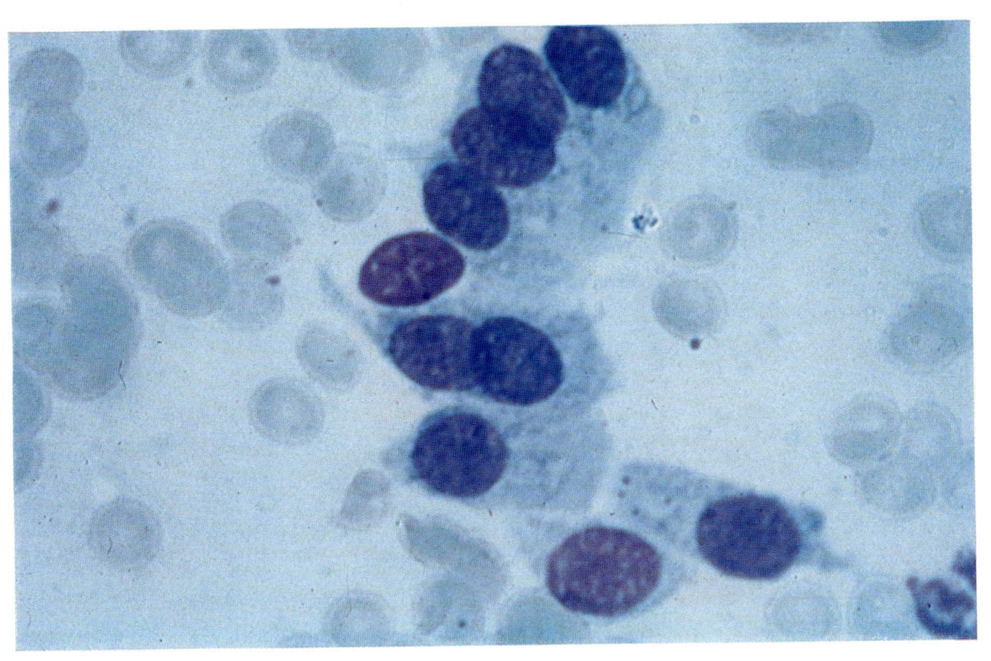

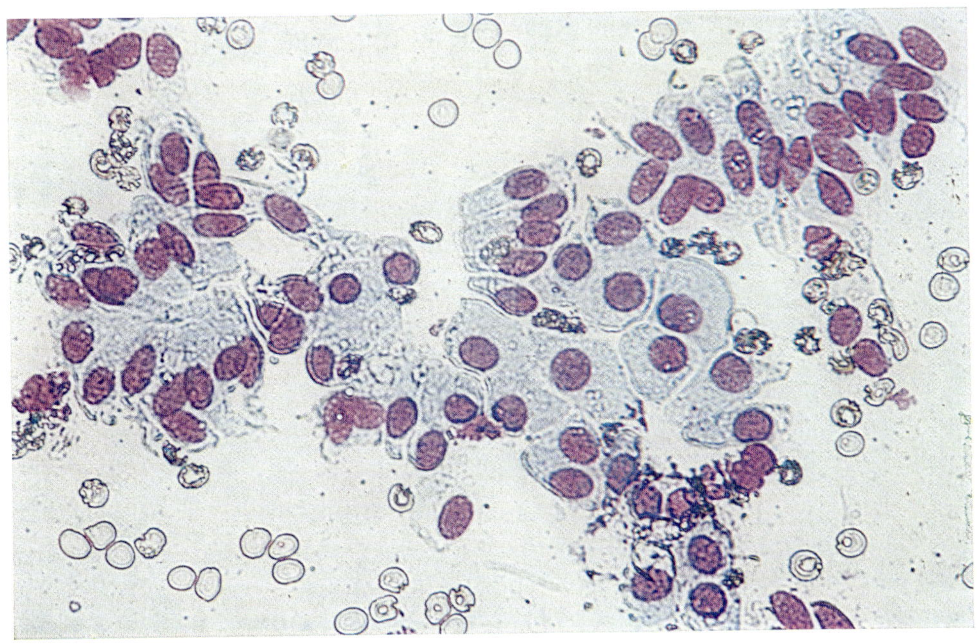

Fig. D.97. — Histologic preparation of the normal ampulla of the ductus deferens of a 29-year-old man. Notice the marked polymorphism and polychromasia of the nuclei of the epithelial mucosa and their loose chromatin pattern and prominent nucleoli, especially in the basal portions of the mucosa (left and middle halves of the picture). In the middle and upper portions of the mucous membrane (right side of the picture), the nuclei are smaller, more uniform, and have a denser chromatin structure (HE, 1,250×, oil immersion).

Fig. D.98. — Marked polymorphism of seminal vesicle cells arising, for the most part, from the ampulla. The large nuclei, rich in chromatin, show an entirely uniform internal structure, polychromasia, and hyperchromasia. The cytoplasm is indistinct (May-Grünwald-Giemsa, 1,000×, oil immersion).

126

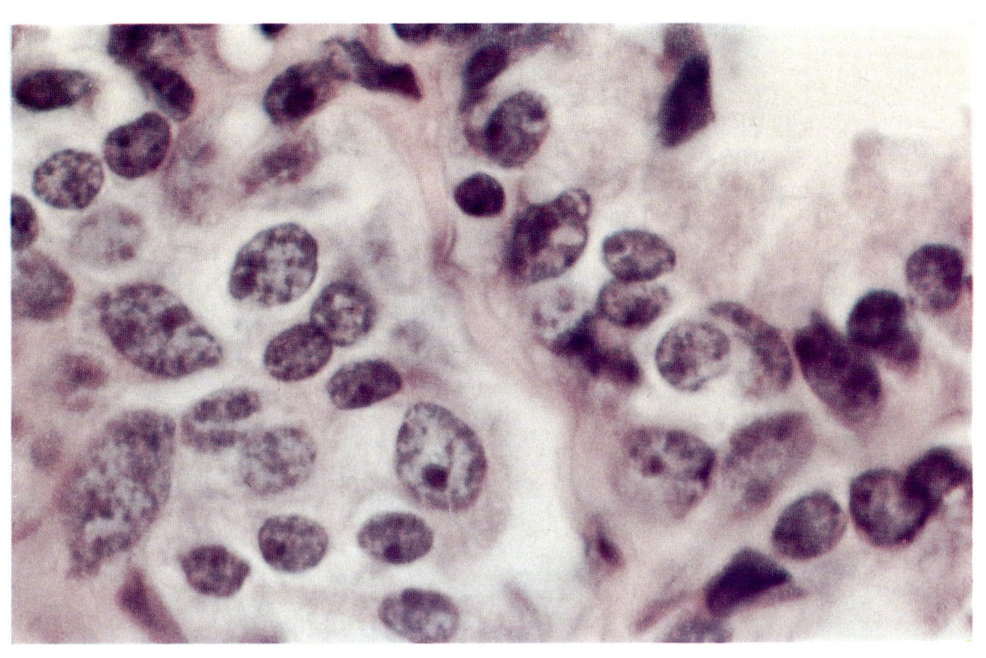

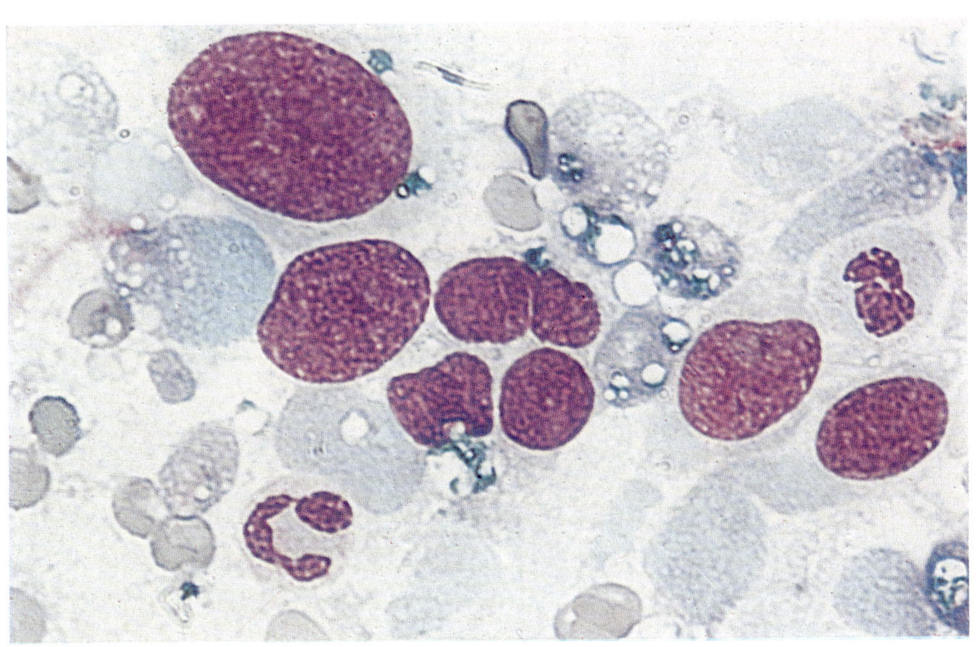

b) Spermatozoa

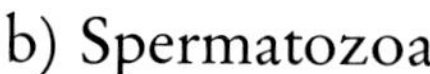

Fig.D.99. – Sheet of prostatic cells surrounded by spermatozoa (May-Grünwald-Giemsa, 400×).

c) Urinary Bladder

Fig.D.100. – Unilayered sheet of normal, uniform prostatic cells on the right. On the left, bladder cells. The transitional epithelium of the urinary bladder is recognized by the greater nuclear size and polymorphism. The basophilic staining of the cytoplasm and sheet pattern are clearly shown (May-Grünwald-Giemsa, 250×).

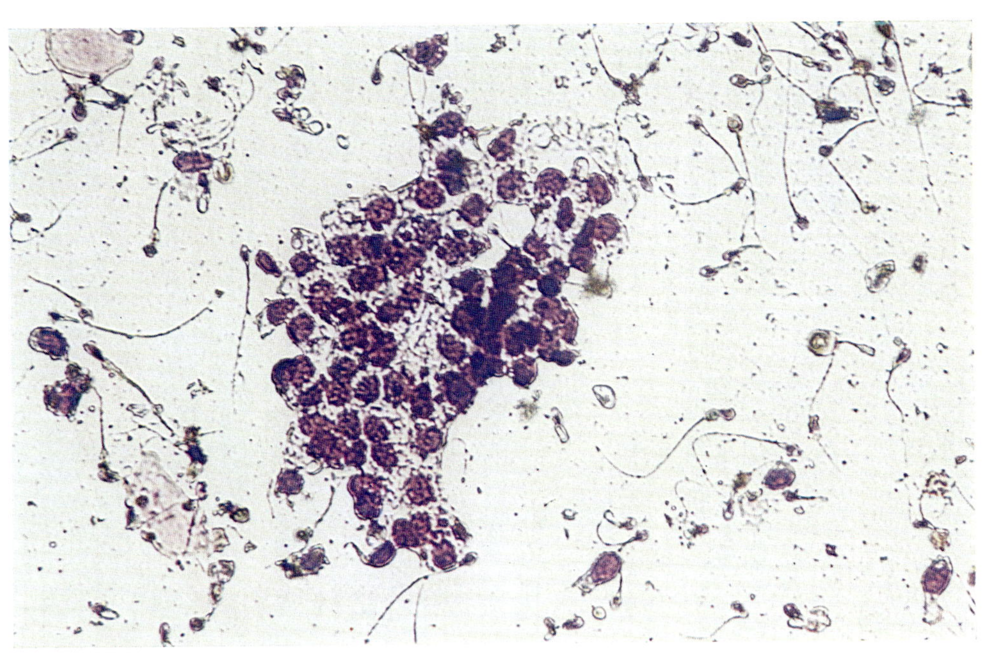

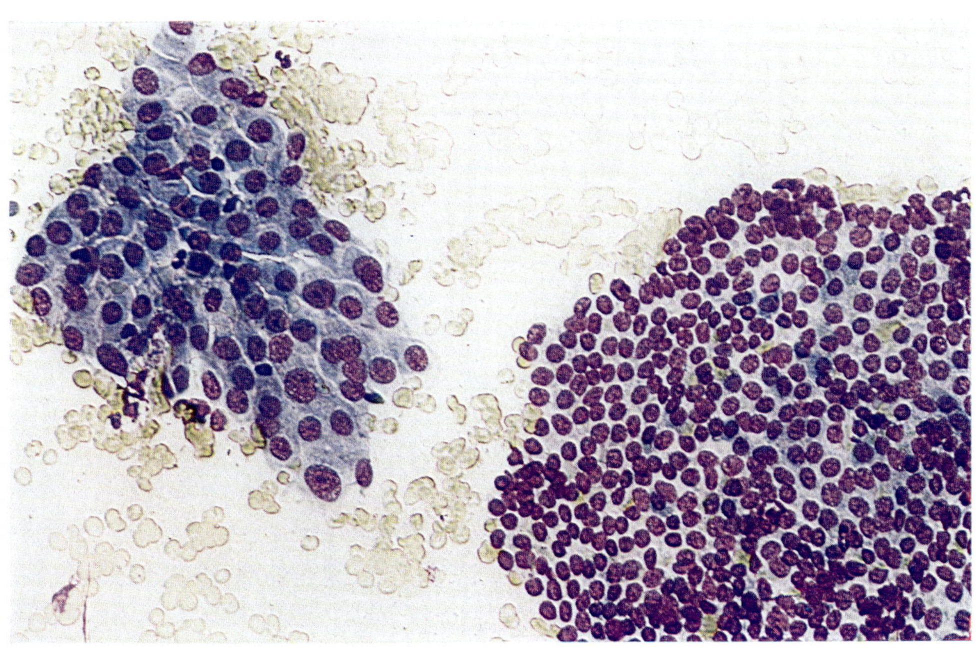

Fig. D.101. – Sheet of transitional epithelial cells from the urinary bladder. The cells have larger nuclei than prostatic cells, and for the most part the cytoplasm is uniformly basophilic with distinct cell borders. There are no signs of malignancy (May-Grünwald-Giemsa, 400×).

d) Rectum

Fig. D.102. – Cylindrical epithelium from the rectum. The elongated oval nuclei having loose internal structure and abundant cytoplasm with focal granular vacuolation or cytoplasmic inclusions are characteristic (May-Grünwald-Giemsa, 1,000×, oil immersion).

130

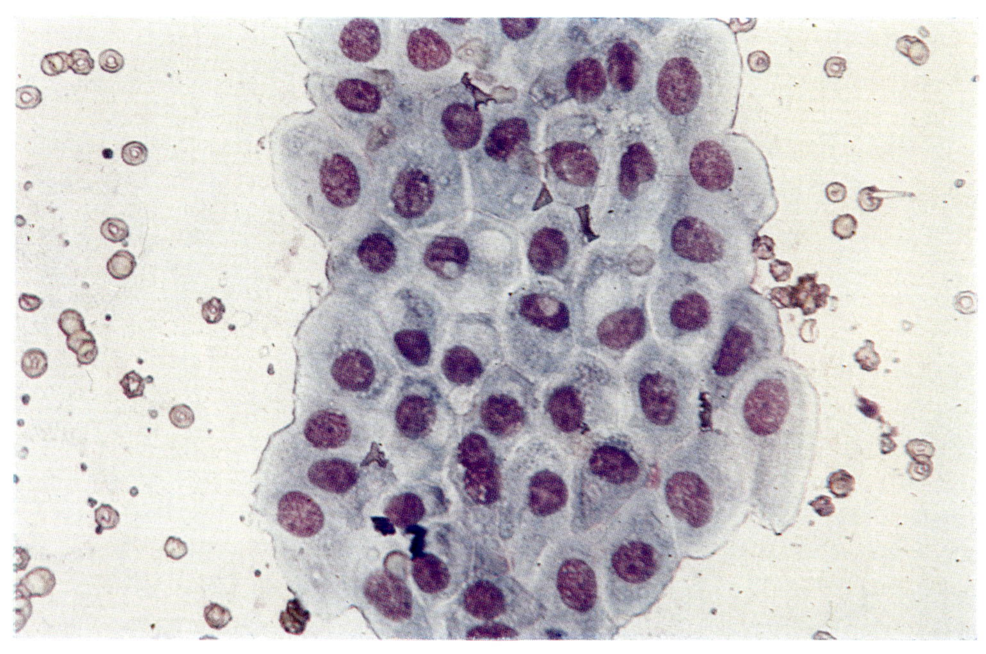

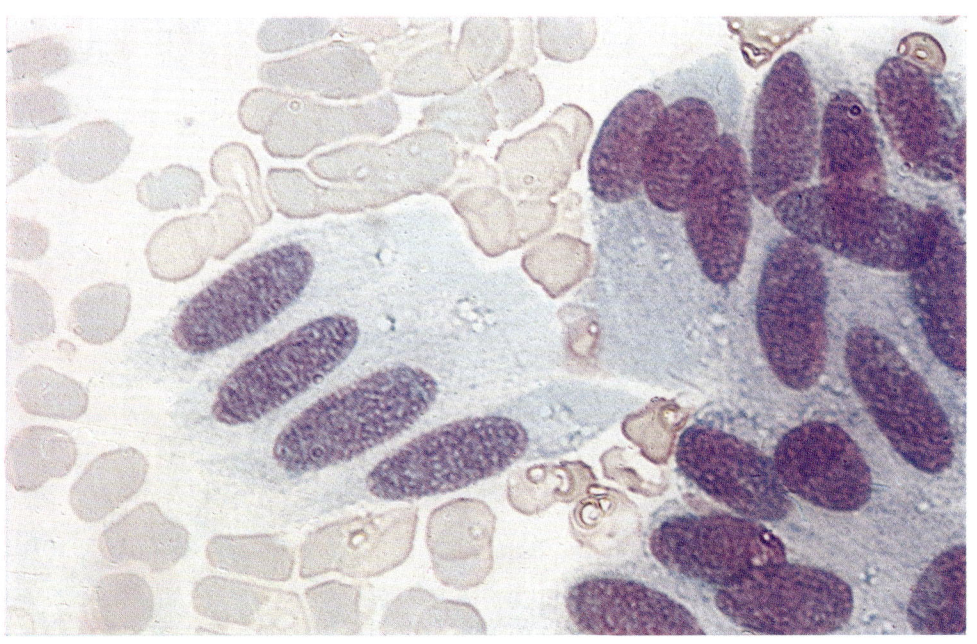

Fig. D.103. − A sheet of prostatic cells lies in the lower left half of the picture and beside it a sheet of cells from the rectum showing the typical cylindrical epithelium and large, oval nuclei. The variation in nuclear size is within normal limits. The cytoplasm is abundant with focal vacuolization (May-Grünwald-Giemsa, 400×).

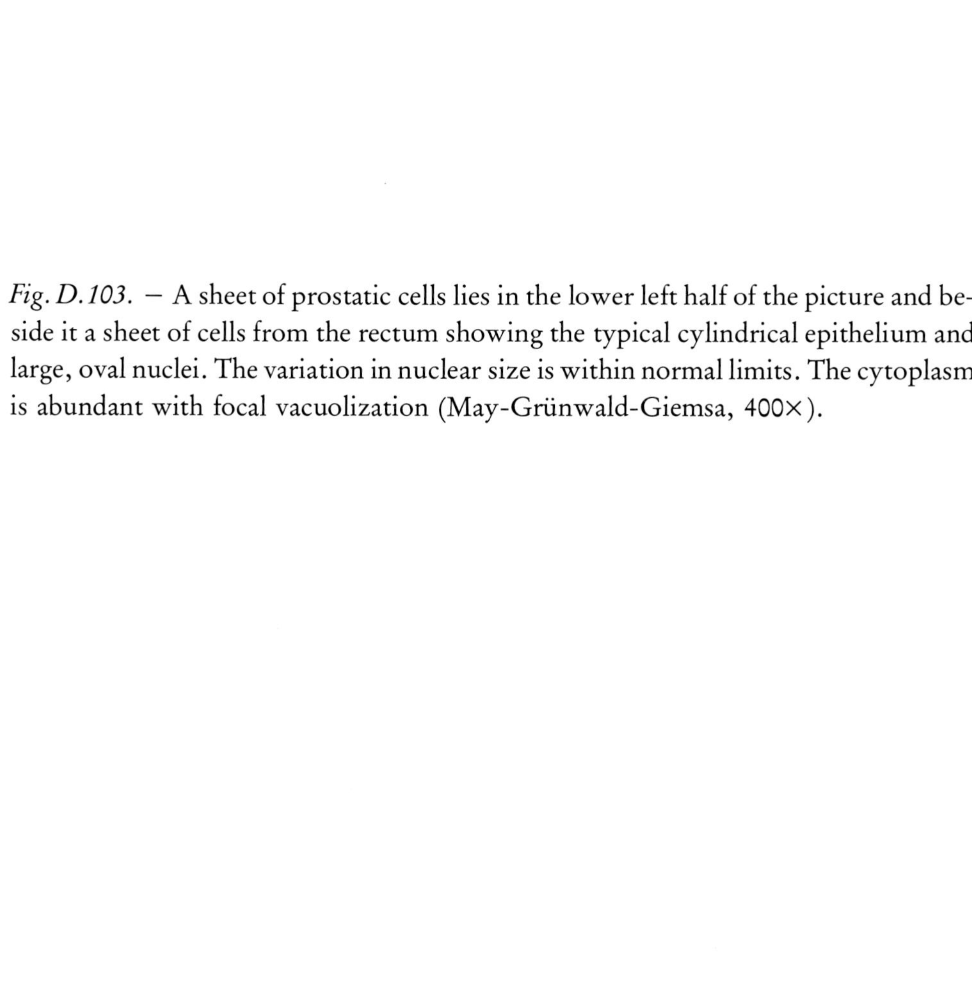

Fig. D.104. − Sheet of rectal cells, many of which overlap. The fine granularity of the cytoplasm is typical. The characteristic goblet shape seen in histologic sections is not apparent in cytologic preparations (May-Grünwald-Giemsa, 1,000×, oil immersion).

132

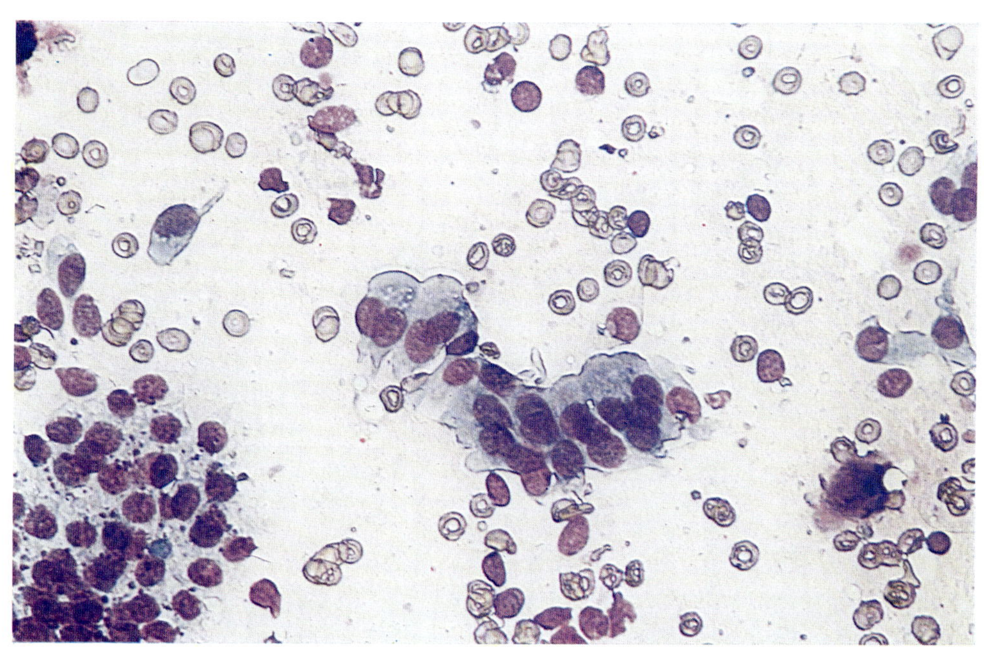

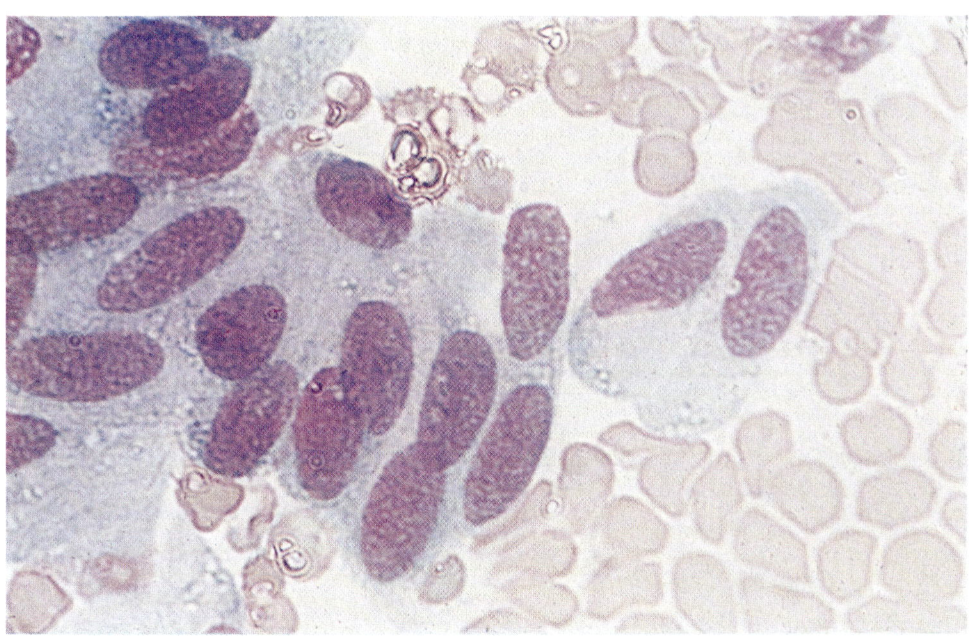

Fig.D.105. – Cylindrical epithelium from the rectum. The internal structure of the nuclei is somewhat dense with distinct hyperchromatic clumping. The cytoplasm is abundant and basophilic (May-Grünwald-Giemsa, 1,000×, oil immersion).

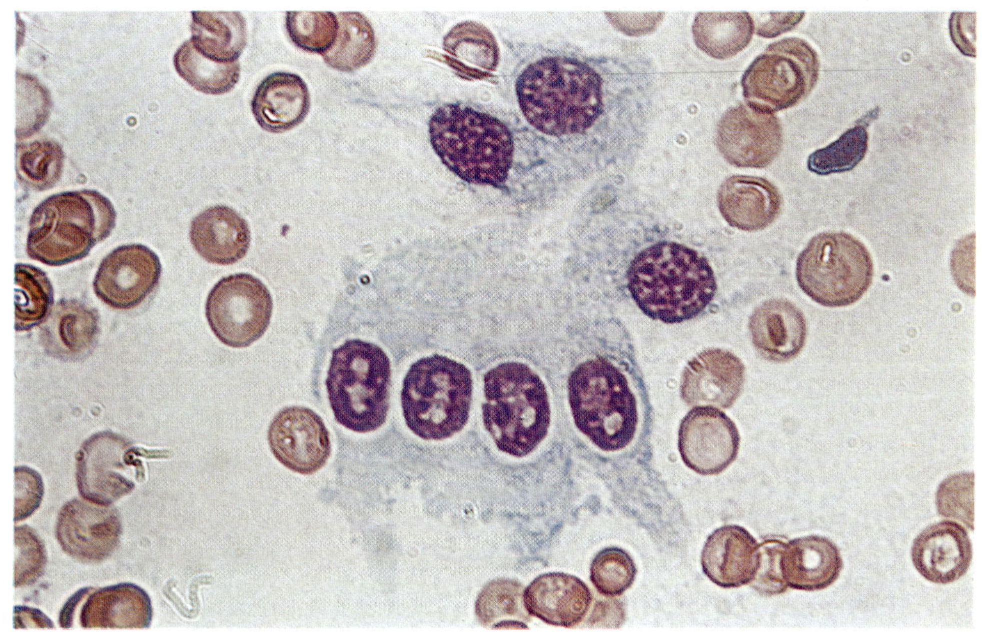

E. References

(1) ANDERSSON, L., JÖNSSON, G., and BRUNK, U.: Puncture biopsy of the prostate in diagnosis of prostatic cancer, Scand. J. Urol. Nephrol. *1:* 227, 1967.

(2) CHU, E. W., and HOJE, R. C.: The clinician and the cytopathologist evaluate fine needle aspiration cytology, Acta Cytol. *17:* 413, 1973.

(3) COMAN, D. R.: Decreased mutual adhesiveness; property of cells from squamous cell carcinoma, Cancer Res. *4:* 625, 1944.

(4) ESPOSTI, P. L.: Cytologic diagnosis of prostatic tumors with the aid of transrectal aspiration biopsy, Acta Cytol. *10:* 182, 1966.

(5) ESPOSTI, P. L.: Cytologic malignancy grading of prostatic carcinoma by transrectal aspiration biopsy, Scand. J. Urol. Nephrol. *5:* 199, 1971.

(6) ESPOSTI, P. L., FRANZÉN, S., and ZAJICEK, J.: The Aspiration Biopsy Smear, in Koss, L. G. (ed.): *Diagnostic Cytology and Its Histopathologic Bases* (2d ed.; Philadelphia: Lippincott, 1968), pp. 565–596.

(7) FAUL, P., KLOSTERHALFEN, H., and SCHMIEDT, E.: Erfahrungen mit der Feinnadelbiopsie der Prostata, Urologe A *10:* 120, 1971.

(8) FERGUSON, R. S.: Prostatic neoplasms: Their diagnosis by needle puncture and aspiration, Amer. J. Surg. *9:* 507, 1930.

(9) FERGUSON, R. S.: Diagnosis and treatment of early carcinoma of the prostate, J. Urol. *37:* 774, 1937.

(10) FERGUSON, J. D., and FRANKS, L. M.: The response of prostatic carcinoma to oestrogen treatment, Brit. J. Surg. *40:* 2, 1953.

(11) FRANK, I. N.: A cytologic evaluation of the prostatic smear in carcinoma of the prostate, J. Urol. *73:* 128, 1955.

(12) FRANK, I. N., and SCOTT, W. W.: The cytodiagnosis of prostatic carcinoma: A follow-up study, J. Urol. *79:* 983, 1958.

(13) FRANZÉN, S., GIERTZ, G., and ZAJICEK, J.: Cytological diagnosis of prostatic tumours by transrectal aspiration biopsy, Brit. J. Urol. *32:* 193, 1960.

(14) KAUFMANN, J. J., ROSENTHAL, M., and GOODWIN, W. E.: Methods of diagnosis of carcinoma of the prostate, J. Urol. *72:* 450, 1954.

(15) KOSS, L. G.: *Diagnostic Cytology* (2d ed.; Philadelphia, Toronto: Lippincott, 1968).

(16) McCUTCHEON, M., COMAN, D. R., and MOORE, F. B.: Studies on invasiveness of cancer; adhesiveness of malignant cells in various human adenocarcinomas, Cancer *1:* 460, 1948.

(17) PAPANICOLAOU, G. N., and TRAUT, H. F.: *Diagnosis of Uterine Cancer by the Vaginal Smear* (New York: Commonwealth Fund, 1943).

(18) RICH, A. R.: On the frequency of occurrence of occult carcinoma of the prostate, J. Urol. *33:* 215, 1935.

(19) SCHUBERT, G. E., ZIEGLER, H., and VÖLTER, D.: Vergleichende histologische und cytologische Untersuchungen der Prostata unter besonderer Berücksichtigung östrogeninduzierter Veränderungen, Verh. Dtsch. Ges. Path. *57:* 315, 1973.

(20) SIKA, J. V., and LINDQUIST, H. D.: Relationship of needle biopsy diagnosis of prostate to clinical signs of prostatic cancer: An evaluation of 300 cases, J. Urol. *89:* 737, 1963.

(21) STAEHLER, W., VÖLTER, D., and ZIEGLER, H.: Die Alterserkrankungen der Prostata im Rahmen der Vorsorgeuntersuchung, Med. Welt 24 (N. F.): 115, 1973.

(22) VÖLTER, D., and ZIEGLER, H.: Die Bedeutung der Cytologie für die Diagnostik der Prostatitis, Med. Welt 24 (N. F.): 356, 1973.

(23) VÖLTER, D., and ZIEGLER, H.: Prostataadenom und -carcinom, Phlebol. Proktol. *2:* 247, 1973.

(24) ZIEGLER, H., and VÖLTER, D.: Die cytologische Diagnostik der Prostatitis, Urologe A *12:* 123, 1973.

(25) ZIEGLER, H., VÖLTER, D., and SCHUBERT, G. E.: Histologische und cytologische Untersuchungen von Prostatagewebe, Verh. Dtsch. Ges. Urol. *24:* 263, 1972.

140